LEADING-EDGE COGNITIVE DISORDERS RESEARCH

LEADING-EDGE COGNITIVE DISORDERS RESEARCH

JAMES P. TSAI
EDITOR

Nova Science Publishers, Inc.
New York

For permission to use material from this book please contact us:
Telephone 631-231-7269; Fax 631-231-8175
Web Site: http://www.novapublishers.com

LIBRARY OF CONGRESS CATALOGING-IN-PUBLICATION DATA

Leading-edge cognitive disorders research / James P. Tsai (editor).
p. ; cm.
Includes bibliographical references and index.
ISBN-13: 978-1-60021-843-9 (hardcover)
ISBN-10: 1-60021-843-1 (hardcover)
1. Cognition disorders. I. Tsai, James P.
[DNLM: 1. Delirium, Dementia, Amnestic, Cognitive Disorders--etiology. 2. Delirium, Dementia, Amnestic, Cognitive Disorders--diagnosis. 3. Delirium, Dementia, Amnestic, Cognitive Disorders--therapy. 4. Research Design. WM 140 L434 2008]
RC553.C64L43 2008
616.80072--dc22 2007032042

Published by Nova Science Publishers, Inc. ✣ New York

CONTENTS

PREFACE

This new book presents important recent research on congitive disorders which are disturbances in the mental process related to thinking, reasoning, and judgment. They include delirium, dementia, and other cognitive disorders. Cognition includes the domains of attention, memory, language, gnosis, visuospatial function, praxis, and executive function, and is traditionally distinguished from the emotions or "feelings." Cognitive disorders may disturb one domain specifically, as in a selective impairment of memory (amnesia) or language (aphasia), or, more often, a combination of deficits, as in mental retardation and dementia.

Chapter 1 - The most recent research on cognition in aging reveals the presence of cognitive deficits long before the clinical diagnosis of dementia can be made. Individuals presenting with Mild Cognitive Impairment (MCI) are now considered to be in a transitional state between normal aging and mild dementia. Given that early treatments (e.g. cognitive stimulation techniques, pharmacological treatment, etc.) can potentially improve their prognosis and quality of life, the detection of MCI patients and the accurate prediction of their subsequent clinical evolution is of major importance. Consequently, there is an increased need for an efficient cognitive screening measure which will succeed in fulfilling these special requirements. The goal of this chapter is to critically review the available data on the ability of some of the most popular screening tests to identify individuals with MCI. Original data on the diagnostic validity of the Mattis Dementia Rating Scale is also presented.

Chapter 2 – The authors propose that the mode of action of polyunsaturated essential fatty acids (PUFA) results from its effect in stabilizing and protecting the structure and functions of the neuronal membrane. PUFA's many effects include brain physiology that modulate pain, thermoregulation and sleep, and brain biochemistry that affects brain neurotransmitters, cholesterol, myelin, and cortisone. Related CNS disorders include Alzheimer's dementia, epilepsy and multiple sclerosis, which are notable for the disruption of normal cognitive behaviors. The authors further propose that not only will a deficiency in brain PUFA will lead to cognitive deficits, but that supplementation of PUFA can rehabilitate many of the consequent deficits. In addition, they conclude that the *ratio* of the two types of PUFA, viz. omega-3 and omega-6 with an optimum ratio of 1:4, is in fact even more important than the absolute level of either.

Chapter 3 - The concept of frailty, a decrease in physical function and increasing vulnerability to morbidity and death, is central to the biological study of aging. Genetics, epigenetics, free radicals, aging, disease, and cellular bioenergetics have all been identified as causative elements in frailty. Study of these elements, and their relations, may allow us to develop dynamic models of the age related emergence of physical frailty at the population level. A phenotype has been defined for physical frailty. An area where frailty is less completely studied is the central nervous system (CNS) where a phenotype has not been developed for cognitive "frailty". The authors attempt to develop such a model by examining the effects of loss of neuronal energetic capacity with age.

To develop a model of frailty in the CNS the ability to parametrically describe changes in neuronal frailty and mortality must be examined in the context of the properties of cellular processes involved in energy production. Processes whose contribution to CNS frailty are to be examined include a) shortening of the telomere by oxidative stress, b) cellular bioenergetics involving mitochondrial enzyme, membrane and matrix structure, c) select genes silencing the expression of specific proteins, and d) genomic and non-genomic thyroid hormone (*Triiodothyronine (T3))* regulation of mitochondrial structure and function, genesis and cell growth and differentiation. The role of environmental stressors, such as ionizing radiation (IR), in modifying certain rate parameters of cellular bioenergetics may suggests ways to better study and describe such mechanisms in humans.

Chapter 4 - With increasing emphasis on early diagnosis of Alzheimer Disease (AD), clinical research has focused on the identification of risk factors that may be modified at a preclinical and early clinical stage of dementing disorders. Prevalence and incidence of different predementia syndromes vary as a result of different diagnostic criteria, as well as different sampling and assessment procedures. Particular interest in Mild Cognitive Impairment (MCI) arises from the fact that MCI is thought to be a prodromal phase and therefore highly predictive of subsequent AD. Furthermore, many of the risk factors for cerebrovascular disease (CVD) and vascular dementia, including serum total cholesterol, hypertension, atherosclerosis, and apolipoprotein E (APOE) genotype have also been shown to increase the risk of AD. Both vascular factors and APOE ε4 allele have been associated with higher risk of AD. Some recent studies suggested further that CVD or vascular factors increased the risk of conversion of MCI to dementia. Furthermore, depressive symptoms have been associated with cognitive decline and dementia, but the nature of the temporal relationship remains controversial. In fact, studies have ranged from correlating depressive symptoms with subsequent cognitive decline or dementia, cognitive decline or dementia with subsequent depression, to no association between the two. The principal objectives of this chapter were to examine how we might better integrate the varied perspectives on associations among depression, MCI and other predementia syndromes, and cognitive decline and to illuminate the common or distinct mechanisms involved in these associations.

Chapter 5 - In this chapter the authors critically review and discuss methodological questions related to research on cognitive disorders. Research on this area is challenging due to the complexity of functions studied and to the numerous variables implicated. First they revisit the concept of cognition as a mediated (semiotic) and systemic activity. Accordingly, every cognitive act is carried out by a functional network of interconnected mental operations and their processing brain regions, each region belonging to various partly overlapped networks. Therefore, the result of a local lesion is not an isolated symptom but a syndrome, and the best neuropsychological approach is an analysis based on appropriate tests to disclose double dissociations and, in this way, to provide clues to brain-behavior relationships. This approach takes into account the influence of task relevant variables (confounders) related to the patient (e.g., age, education, humor state), to the lesion (size, etiology, acute versus chronic, focal versus diffuse), and to the tests and testing conditions (ecological validity, instructions, examiner's experience, "noise"), which need to be controlled and reckoned in multivariate statistical analyses. Other controversial issues such as single and double dissociations, single-case versus group studies, and the lesion method are also examined. At the end, the authors illustratively bring up methodological problems of current cognitive research on early multiple sclerosis and medial temporal lobe epilepsy.

Chapter 6 - There are few criminal offences capable of stirring up as much public anger and disgust as child molestation. Despite the media fuelled public perception that child molesters (CMs) cannot be treated, research into the cognition of CMs is suggesting that the authors may be able to challenge some of the belief structures of these individuals and thus change their behavior patterns. Attempts to discover why some people molest children are paramount to delivering effective treatment programs. In this chapter, the authors will provide an overview of the main research methodologies and theories that have been developed over the past two decades to investigate the cognitive distortions of CMs and consider how empirical research may inform treatment programs.

It is perhaps not surprising that the cognition of CMs (i.e., what they think and believe), has become central to both research and treatment programs over the last two decades since virtually all contemporary theories of child molestation highlight the importance of cognition. The role of cognitive distortions in particular has been suggested as fundamental to the etiology and treatment of child sexual abuse. The underlying assumption is that CMs' thinking is distorted or different from non-molesters in distinct and important ways. It is these distortions in thinking that the authors intend to focus upon in this chapter.

In: Leading-Edge Cognitive Disorders Research
Editor: James P. Tsai, pp. 1-4
ISBN: 978-1-60021-843-9

Expert Commentary A

MISUNDERSTANDINGS SURROUNDING THE TREATMENT OF JUVENILE DELINQUENCY

Lauren C. Gudonis and Peter R. Giancola[1]
University of Kentucky, USA

Despite the numerous social and economic costs of juvenile delinquency to our society, there exists a general consensus within the field that therapeutic interventions for this population are generally ineffective (Hammersley, Reid, and Minkes, 2006; Chitsabesan, and Bailey, 2006; Tate, Reppucci, and Mulvey, 1995). Although some studies hint at positive treatment results (Caldwell, Skeem, Salekin, Van-Rybroek, 2006), many of the antisocial behaviors often associated with juvenile delinquency appear resistant to intervention at long-term follow-ups (for a review, see Tarolla et al., 2002). This pessimism surrounding treatment of juvenile delinquency is understandable. The specific characteristics that define this population (i.e. impulsivity, deceitfulness, co-morbidity with substance use and other psychological disorders) are often stable and extremely resistant to change. Regardless of any reported failures in treatment response, however, it erroneous to conclude this population is *untreatable* based on the empirical treatment evidence alone.

Perhaps the lack of treatment effectiveness is not a function of this population in need, but instead a result of poorly implemented, narrowly focused, and theoretically inadequate treatments. For example, one major issue that plagues treatment efficacy is the development of treatments based on "blind" direct translation of theory. An example of this is the implementation of standard cognitive-behavioral treatments. Over the years, a vast amount of research has uncovered deficits in both intellective and non-intellective cognitive functioning among delinquents. Juvenile delinquents often present with poor problem solving skills, ineffective or problematic coping skills, low executive functioning, and distorted thinking styles. In response, one of the most common interventions employed in both forensic and community settings are cognitive-behavioral treatments (CBT) for these troubled adolescents. These treatments focus on the identification and modification of maladaptive thoughts and

[1] Corresponding Author: Peter Giancola, Department of Psychology, University of Kentucky, Lexington, KY, 40506-0044 or email to PETER@UKY.EDU.

behaviors to change thinking styles, interpersonal skills, communication, and problem-solving ability. Some statistical support for the effectiveness of this treatment mode has been established and should be recognized. For example, some meta-analytic studies have found that CBT treatments are effective in improving social problem-solving skills and impulsivity among adolescents (Garrett, 1985; Lipsey and Wilson, 1998). Despite such optimistic findings, however, the improvements are rarely maintained beyond the setting in which the treatment was implemented. Moreover, gains are often not maintained when evaluated at 1-year follow-ups.

Perhaps this lack of permanent change implies that translation from research on cognitive deficiencies directly to cognitive treatments to alter such deficits is a mistake. One possible oversight is that the delinquent population itself may not be accurate observers of their feelings and/or cognitions (Rohde et al., 2004). Moreover, traditional developmental theory suggests the abstract thinking abilities and operational processes of young adolescents are often limited and not fully developed until the later years. Yet the process of CBT requires exactly this; the ability to scientifically evaluate one's own dysfunctional thoughts, interpersonal patterns, and inadequate communication styles in order to change them. The techniques of CBT itself may be one barrier in producing long-term meaningful changes in juvenile delinquents.

The direct translation of basic research into treatment development is also apparent in therapies that employ peer group counseling techniques. A well-established risk factor associated with adolescent delinquency is the association with deviant peers, rejection by peers, and bullying by peers. Adolescents exposed to negative peer influences are placed at a greater risk for the development of aggressive behavior, antisocial attitudes, drug use, and other types of criminal behavior. One type of treatment response to reduce the weight of this risk factor that has received some attention is the peer group counseling environment. Employed often within the juvenile justice system, the technique involves the immersion of delinquent peers with each other to encourage the promotion of honest communication, problem-solving, respect, and a variety of other prosocial interaction styles and attitudes. Unfortunately, the ability of such treatments to elicit substantive change in problem adolescents has been minimal. Despite the evidence that supports peer influence as a prominent risk factor for delinquency, there is little empirical evidence that suggests immersing delinquent peers with each other will promote prosocial behavior. If anything, the research suggests that association with delinquent peers allows for greater exposure to antisocial behavior, thereby enriching criminal versatility and skill. Again, it is suggested that creating treatment modalities that directly address or try to modify a single, empirically established risk factor may be a premature attempt at a "quick fix" solution for a problem whose complexity and resistance should not be overlooked. Moreover, the relation between a single risk factor and the later development of delinquency is rarely linear and direct. Interactions between multiple risk and protective factors serve as a more comprehensive and practical basis for thinking about treatment possibilities.

The above examples are just two of many therapeutic interventions that place a heavy focus on changing single risk factors in an attempt to elicit long-lasting behavior change. It should be noted that the problems and restrictions addressed thus far are not necessarily innovative or unknown to the field. However, most of these problems within the treatment literature are placed simply in the "limitation" section as methodological oversights or study constraints. If researchers instead incorporate these acknowledged limitations into improved theories and methods, than perhaps treatments for juvenile delinquency can more effectively reduce long-term problem behaviors.

Finally, it is argued that many current treatments fail to appreciate the extreme heterogeneity found within the broad classification of juvenile delinquency. Risk factors that have been established for the development of delinquency and later violent or offending behavior are numerous. They occur on multiple levels, and involve the interaction of complex layers beginning with individual child factors and culminating in societal factors. Difficult temperament, impulsive personality traits, poor parenting practices, poor academic performance, rejection by peers, and media portrayal of violence provides just a sampling of the myriad of risk factors that needs to be considered before successful interventions can be developed (for excellent comprehensives reviews of this topic, see the following: Loeber and Farrington, 2000; Tarolla et al., 2002) The important take-home message within this research is that no two adolescents will present with identical "blueprints" for the development of delinquency. Every individual causal pathway is different, even within children who come from the same home environment. Although common risk factors may present in many delinquents, treatments that focus on modifying only a single risk factor are theoretically meaningless. Ignoring the diverse treatment needs of this group will result in therapeutic interventions that will likely continue to produce short-term, artificial improvements.

REFERENCES

Caldwell, M., Skeem, J., Salekin, R., and VanRybroek, G. (2006). Treatment response of adolescent offenders with psychopathy features: A 2-year follow-up. *Criminal Justice and Behavior, 33,* 571-596.

Chitsabesan, P. and Bailey, S. (2006). Mental health, educational and social needs of young offenders in custody and in the community. *Current Opinion in Psychiatry, 4,* 355-360.

Garrett, C.J. (1985). Effects of residential treatment on adjudicated delinquents: a meta-analysis. *Journal of Research in Crime and Delinquency, 22*, 671-714.

Hammersley, R., Reid, M., and Minkes, J. (2006). Treatment for substance use problems among young offenders: Difficulties and dilemmas for implementation and evaluation in the UK. *Educational and Clinical Psychology, 23*, 41-51.

Lipsey, M.W., and Wilson, D.B. (1998). Effective intervention for serious juvenile offenders: a synthesis of research. In: R. Loeber, and D.P. Farrington (Eds.), *Serious and violent juvenile offenders: risk factors and successful interventions* (pp. 313-345). Thousand Oaks, CA: Sage.

Loeber, R., and Farrington, D.P. (2000). Young children who commit crime: Epidemiology, developmental origins, risk factors, early interventions, and policy implications. *Development and Psychopathology,* 12, 737-762.

Rohde, P., Jorgensen, J.S., Seeley, J.R., and Mace, D.E. (2004). Pilot evaluation of the coping course: A cognitive-behavioral intervention to enhance coping skills in incarcerated youth. *Journal of the American Academy of Adolescent Psychiatry, 43,* 669-676.

Tarolla, S.M., Wagner, E.F., Rabinowitz, J., and Tubman, J.G. (2002). Understanding and treating juvenile offenders: A review of current knowledge and future directions.

Aggression and Violent Behavior, 7, 125-143.Tate, D.C., Reppucci, N., and Mulvey, E.P. (1995). Violent juvenile delinquents: treatment effectiveness and implications for future action. *American Psychologists, 50,* 777-781.

In: Leading-Edge Cognitive Disorders Research
Editor: James P. Tsai, pp. 5-8

ISBN: 978-1-60021-843-9

Expert Commentary B

SCREENING TESTS FOR DETECTION OF MILD COGNITIVE IMPAIRMENT

Evelyne Matteau[a], Martine Simard[a], Léonie Jean[a], and Yves Turgeon[b]

[a]École de psychologie, Université Laval, and Centre de recherche Université Laval Robert-Giffard, Quebec city, Quebec, Canada.

[b]Department of Psychology and Restigouche Memory Centre, Campbellton, New-Brunswick, Canada

The results discussed in the chapter entitled Detection of Mild Cognitive Impairment Using Cognitive Screening Tests: A Critical Review and Preliminary Data on the Mattis Dementia Rating Scale, showed that some of the most used cognitive screening tests were capable to detect, to a certain degree, the preclinical state of dementia, especially dementia of the Alzheimer's type. However, the review has also underlined some critical points that need to be further developed in the domain study of Mild Cognitive Impairment (MCI).

First, it has been emphasized that neuropsychological screening measures should cover a wide range of cognitive functions in order to tap those reportedly impaired long before the clinical diagnosis of dementia can be made. Ideally, the episodic memory examination shall be designed in order to distinguish the different processes such as encoding, consolidation and retrieval that could be altered in MCI. This exhaustive evaluation of memory processes is not only important for the diagnosis of amnesic-MCI (A-MCI) but also for the prognosis of future evolution. Indeed, it is likely that encoding / consolidation failures would lead to Alzheimer's disease (AD), a cortical dementia, and that retrieval problem would rather indicate a frontal-subcortical dysfunction (Traykov et al., 2005). Similarly, the evaluation of executive functions, along with that of memory, is particularly important since a dysexecutive syndrome may underscore the presence of a different neurodegenerative pathology such as fronto-temporal and vascular subcortical dementias (Zanetti et al., 2006). The examination of multiple cognitive domains thus allows to study the various MCI subtypes that could evolve to different forms of dementia. Along with other authors (Chong and Sahadevan, 2005), we believe that screening measures of cognition may be different from one clinical setting to the other.. Nevertheless, they should have good psychometric qualities as well as sensitivity / specificity values that permit to calculate likelihood ratios. Moreover, normative data should be available that take into account the cultural background, and at least the age and education level of populations under study.

Recently, Petersen and O'Brien (2006) have argued that MCI is not a neuropsychological diagnosis that should be based on a single cutoff score, and that it relies ultimately on clinical judgment. The clinician attempting to identify individuals at risk to evolve towards dementia must first exclude all other potential causes of cognitive impairments (e.g. metabolic changes, medication side effects, etc.), and interpret changes in cognitive status in the context of each individual's history. A decline from a previous level of functioning should be established by testing or using the report of a significant informant prior to the diagnosis of impairment (Collie and Maruff, 2002). In such conditions, at least one follow-up data collection is necessary to improve MCI diagnosis specificity.

Apart from cognitive functioning, several predictors of progression are currently studied. Research on biomarkers like ApoEε4 genotype and cerebral imaging have provided some interesting results (Chetelat et al., 2005). However, these results need to be expanded and replicated in order to better know about their sensitivity and specificity to detect dementia syndromes. The presence or absence of functional impairments in complex versus basic activities of daily living in the preclinical state of dementia also needs to be clarified (Perneczky et al., 2006).

Moreover, we believe that the assessment of the predictive value of behavioral and psychological symptoms have been neglected to date, perhaps because of the current conceptualization of MCI as a neurocognitive disorder. Almost all patients suffering from dementia syndromes will, at one moment or another, experiencing symptoms such as disorders of thought, content, mood or behaviour (Finkel, Costa e Silva, Cohen, Miller, and Sartorius, 1996). Recent prevalence studies have demonstrated that neuropsychiatric symptoms are also part of the MCI condition (Lyketsos et al., 2002; Tatsch et al., 2006). For example, depression and / or apathy are frequently seen in early AD (Lyketsos et al., 2002), dementia with Lewy bodies (Simard, van Reekum, and Cohen, 2000), and preclinical AD (Jean, Simard, van Reekum, and Clarke, 2005). In addition, some data suggested that a REM Sleep Behavior Disorder may appear several years before the development of synucleopathy diseases such as dementia with Lewy bodies and Parkinson's disease with dementia (McKeith et al., 2005). Studying these particular symptoms provides the opportunity to better understand brain-behavior relationships (Lyketsos et al., 2002). Consequently, psychological and behavioral symptoms prior to, or concomitant with cognitive deficits, can be considered as potential markers for the MCI diagnosis.

When sufficient data on various risk factors will be available, more detailed MCI subtypes criteria will be described that will reflect the best components of an interdisciplinary approach. In function of these optimal criteria, construction and testing of simple algorithms that can be easily applied by clinicians may greatly improve predictive validity of MCI.

Finally, once the diagnosis of MCI will be made with confidence, the issue of early treatment should seriously be addressed given the difficult consequences for MCI individuals. Pharmaceutical agents may delay or even improve the progression of cognitive impairment (Petersen et al., 2005; Simard, Van Reekum, and Suvajac, 2000). Techniques such as cognitive remediation and/or training are certainly another useful therapeutic avenue to be investigated. The most adequate method to assess a response to treatment in patients with

MCI is neuropsychological testing (Luis, Loewenstein, Acevedo, Barker, and Duara, 2003). In order to do so, we need valid instruments, available in several alternative forms, and sensitive to potential changes in cognitive functioning. Because the patient's and his caregiver's perception of difficulties may affect self-esteem and mood, the subjective appreciation of the patient treated and his/her surroundings should also be considered as a measure of improvement. Following a better recognition of neuropsychiatric symptoms in MCI, more emotional / psychotherapeutic intervention will be developed in the future.

REFERENCES

Chetelat, G., Eustache, F., Viader, F., De La Sayette, V., Pelerin, A., Mezenge, F., et al. (2005). FDG-PET measurement is more accurate than neuropsychological assessments to predict global cognitive deterioration in patients with mild cognitive impairment. *Neurocase, 11*(1), 14-25.

Chong, M. S., and Sahadevan, S. (2005). Preclinical Alzheimer's disease: diagnosis and prediction of progression. *Lancet Neurology, 4*(9), 576-579.

Collie, A., and Maruff, P. (2002). An analysis of systems of classifying mild cognitive impairment in older people. *Australian and New Zealand Journal of Psychiatry, 36*(1), 133-140.

Finkel, S. I., Costa e Silva, J., Cohen, G., Miller, S., and Sartorius, N. (1996). Behavioral and psychological signs and symptoms of dementia: a consensus statement on current knowledge and implications for research and treatment. *International Psychogeriatrics, 8 Suppl 3*, 497-500.

Jean, L., Simard, M., van Reekum, R., and Clarke, D. E. (2005). Differential cognitive impairment in subjects with geriatric depression who will develop Alzheimer's disease and other dementias: a retrospective study. *International Psychogeriatrics, 17*(2), 289-301.

Luis, C. A., Loewenstein, D. A., Acevedo, A., Barker, W. W., and Duara, R. (2003). Mild cognitive impairment: directions for future research. *Neurology, 61*(4), 438-444.

Lyketsos, C. G., Lopez, O., Jones, B., Fitzpatrick, A. L., Breitner, J., and DeKosky, S. (2002). Prevalence of neuropsychiatric symptoms in dementia and mild cognitive impairment: results from the cardiovascular health study. *Journal of American Medical Association, 288*(12), 1475-1483.

McKeith, I. G., Dickson, D. W., Lowe, J., Emre, M., O'Brien, J. T., Feldman, H., et al. (2005). Diagnosis and management of dementia with Lewy bodies: third report of the DLB Consortium. *Neurology, 65*(12), 1863-1872.

Perneczky, R., Pohl, C., Sorg, C., Hartmann, J., Tosic, N., Grimmer, T., et al. (2006). Impairment of activities of daily living requiring memory or complex reasoning as part of the MCI syndrome. *International Journal of Geriatric Psychiatry, 21*(2), 158-162.

Petersen, R. C., Thomas, R. G., Grundman, M., Bennett, D., Doody, R., Ferris, S., et al. (2005). Vitamin E and donepezil for the treatment of mild cognitive impairment. *New England Journal of Medicine, 352*(23), 2379-2388.

Simard, M., van Reekum, R., and Cohen, T. (2000). A review of the cognitive and behavioral symptoms in dementia with Lewy bodies. *Journal of Neuropsychiatry and Clinical Neurosciences, 12*(4), 425-450.

Simard, M., Van Reekum, R., and Suvajac, B. (2000). Improving cognition, behavior, and function, and slowing disease progression of Alzheimer's disease. *Clinical Geriatrics, 8*(11), 32-58.

Tatsch, M. F., Bottino, C. M., Azevedo, D., Hototian, S. R., Moscoso, M. A., Folquitto, J. C., et al. (2006). Neuropsychiatric symptoms in Alzheimer disease and cognitively impaired, nondemented elderly from a community-based sample in Brazil: prevalence and relationship with dementia severity. *American Journal of Geriatric Psychiatry, 14*(5), 438-445.

Traykov, L., Baudic, S., Raoux, N., Latour, F., Rieu, D., Smagghe, A., et al. (2005). Patterns of memory impairment and perseverative behavior discriminate early Alzheimer's disease from subcortical vascular dementia. *Journal of the Neurological Sciences, 229-230*, 75-79.

Zanetti, M., Ballabio, C., Abbate, C., Cutaia, C., Vergani, C., and Bergamaschini, L. (2006). Mild cognitive impairment subtypes and vascular dementia in community-dwelling elderly people: a 3-year follow-up study. *Journal of American Geriatric Society, 54*(4), 580-586.

In: Leading-Edge Cognitive Disorders Research
Editor: James P. Tsai, pp. 9-58
ISBN: 978-1-60021-843-9

Chapter 1

DETECTION OF MILD COGNITIVE IMPAIRMENT USING COGNITIVE SCREENING TESTS: A CRITICAL REVIEW AND PRELIMINARY DATA ON THE MATTIS DEMENTIA RATING SCALE

Evelyne Matteau*[a]*, Martine Simard*[a,1]*,
***Léonie Jean*[a]*, and Yves Turgeon*[b]**

[a]École de psychologie, Université Laval, and Centre de recherche Université Laval Robert-Giffard, Quebec City, Quebec, Canada.

[b]Department of Psychology and Restigouche Memory Centre, Campbellton, New-Brunswick, Canada

ABSTRACT

The most recent research on cognition in aging reveals the presence of cognitive deficits long before the clinical diagnosis of dementia can be made. Individuals presenting with Mild Cognitive Impairment (MCI) are now considered to be in a transitional state between normal aging and mild dementia. Given that early treatments (e.g. cognitive stimulation techniques, pharmacological treatment, etc.) can potentially improve their prognosis and quality of life, the detection of MCI patients and the accurate prediction of their subsequent clinical evolution is of major importance. Consequently, there is an increased need for an efficient cognitive screening measure which will succeed in fulfilling these special requirements. The goal of this chapter is to critically review the available data on the ability of some of the most popular screening tests to identify individuals with MCI. Original data on the diagnostic validity of the Mattis Dementia Rating Scale (MDRS; Mattis, 1988) is also presented.

---

[1] Address of correspondence: Dr. Martine Simard, Ph.D., École de Psychologie, Pavillon Félix-Antoine Savard, Université Laval, Québec, Québec, G1V 0A6, Canada. E-mail: martine.simard@psy.ulaval.ca; Tel: (418) 656-2131, extension 12193; Fax: (418) 656-3646.

Keywords: Mild Cognitive Impairment, screening test, Mini-Mental State Examination, Alzheimer's Disease Assessment Scale – Cognition, Cambridge Examination for Mental Disorders for the Elderly – Cognition, Mattis Dementia Rating Scale, predictive validity, criterion validity, sensitivity, specificity

INTRODUCTION

Neurodegenerative dementias are typically a problem of old age. According to the Canadian Study of Health and Aging (CSHA) Working Group (2000), the risk of developing dementia doubles for each five-year increase in age after 65 years. Previous prevalence estimates of the CSHA suggested that 8% of all Canadians aged 65 and over met the criteria for dementia. The corresponding figures for AD were 5.1% overall (CSHA, 1994). In the United States, AD affected 4.5 million people in 2000, and this prevalence will increase three-fold in 2050 to 13.2 millions individuals (Hebert, Scherr, Bienias, Bennett, and Evans, 2003). Clearly, these data suggest that dementia, Alzheimer's disease and cognitive impairment are common in the elderly, and have become a major health concern in our modern society.

Dementia is characterized by the presence of generalized and persistent cognitive impairment that (a) represents a change from a previous level of functioning, (b) occurs without a disruption in consciousness, (c) is of sufficient severity to influence daily functioning, (d) cannot be explained by situational stress, and (e) may not be the result of a variety of conditions, some of which may be reversible (Fields, 1998). Memory impairment, in combination with deficits in other areas of cognition such as language, visuo-spatial and executive functions, is considered the hallmark feature of dementia, and especially of Alzheimer's disease (AD), by the National Institute of Neurological and Communicative Disorders and Stroke (NINCDS) and the Alzheimer's Disease and Related Disorders Association (ADRDA) (McKhann et al., 1984), and the Diagnostic and Statistical Manual of Mental Disorders (DSM-IV) diagnostic criteria (American Psychiatric Association, 1994).

The proper care of patients with dementia first requires screening to detect memory and other cognitive impairment, then a detailed evaluation for a diagnosis of dementia, and finally, an assessment in order to elucidate a specific cause of dementia (Gifford and Cummings, 1999). The screening assessment usually represents a preliminary filtering phase that identifies the individuals at increased risk of presenting a particular disorder. Individuals found to be «positive» during screening are then required to undergo further diagnostic evaluation, whereas the individuals found to be «negative» usually are not involved in further assessment (Derogatis and Lynn, 2000). The correct identification of the individuals likely to progress to dementia is of particular importance since pharmacological agents altering the course of progressive neurodegenerative disorders, such as AD, are most effective when administered early in the dementia process (Post, 1999; Simard and Sampson, In press; Simard, Van Reekum, and Suvajac, 2000). Furthermore, the diagnosis of dementia at a preclinical stage may allow therapy to be initiated (e.g. cognitive stimulation techniques), and facilitate the education and support to family members.

Intensive research currently aims at facilitating the detection of dementia at a preclinical level. The Mild Cognitive Impairment (MCI) condition is an intermediate state between normal ageing and mild dementia, and could be considered as the prodrome of AD, and possibly other dementias (Ganguli, Dodge, Shen, and DeKosky, 2004; Luis, Loewenstein, Acevedo, Barker, and Duara, 2003; Petersen, 2004). Three subtypes of clinical presentation are proposed by Petersen et al. (2001) : (a) Amnesic MCI or A-MCI, which involves an isolated memory deficit, (b) Multiple-domain MCI or M-MCI, which consists of a mild alteration of several cognitive functions, and (c) Single non-memory domain MCI or S-MCI, which consists of a significant deficit in a cognitive domain other than memory. In all these conditions, the functional capacities of the individual remain relatively preserved (Petersen et al., 2001). While the A-MCI subtype could represent preclinical AD, other MCI subtypes could be indicators of another etiology such as dementia with Lewy bodies, fronto-tremporal dementia, or a psychiatric, vascular or traumatic condition (Petersen, 2004). The content of this chapter will focus on the MCI condition considered as a prodrome of AD.

Depending on the studies, MCI patients register annual conversion rates to dementia from 10% (Petersen et al., 1999; Yesavage et al., 2002) to 41% (Geslani, Tierney, Herrmann, and Szalai, 2005; Larrieu et al., 2002; Mosconi et al., 2004) compared to annual conversion rates from 0.2% to 3.9% (Canadian Study of Health and Aging Working Group, 2000; Larrieu et al., 2002; Petersen et al., 2001) observed in individuals aged ≤ 80 years old without cognitive deficits at baseline. The detection of patients with MCI and their follow-up are highly recommended by the American Academy of Neurology (Petersen et al., 2001).

Unfortunately, primary health care providers do not identify approximately 77% to 95% of individuals presenting with mild cognitive impairment (Callahan, Hendrie, and Tierney, 1995; Ganguli, Rodriguez et al., 2004). This situation is particularly worrisome given the rapid demographic ageing in Western countries (Benson, Slavin, Tran, Petrella, and Doraiswamy, 2005; Chong and Sahadevan, 2005) and the limited access to health care resources in general, especially for neuropsychological assessment (Milberg, 1996). The increasing prevalence of patients presenting with various cognitive dysfunctions, coupled with the limitations in the available resources to address these problems, underline the need for an efficient screening test. The cognitive screening measure should always be interpreted in the patient's clinical context (e.g. onset of symptoms, evolution, medical background, etc) and never be taken as an equivalent of an exhaustive neuropsychological evaluation. Nevertheless, a good screening test may, in a cost- and time-efficient way, guide the clinician in the correct identification of persons who are more likely to present a disorder, in order to refer those who require a more thorough assessment by specialists such as neuropsychologists, neurologists, psychiatrists and geriatricians. The exhaustive assessments performed by the specialists then determine the extent, type and /or etiology of cognitive impairment (Demakis, Mercury, and Sweet, 2000).

The demonstration of clinical effectiveness of a cognitive measure in a given context refers, in psychometric terms, to the criterion-validating procedures (Anastasi and Urbina, 1997). Criterion validity is divided into two categories: concurrent validity and predictive validity. Concurrent validity establishes the correlation between a test score and another external variable which is measured at the same moment but is independent from the performance of the test being validated (Franzen, 2000). Neurophysiological measures are an interesting way to get information about concurrent validity of a neuropsychological test (Franzen, 2000). Because the focus of this chapter is on cognition, this particular aspect of criterion validity will not be discussed further. The present chapter will instead cover studies assessing concurrent validity using group membership as the criterion.

A second category of criterion validity, predictive validity, provides useful information on a test by relating the actual performance on the test to a future outcome (considered as the criterion) (Anastasi and Urbina, 1997; Franzen, 2000). Since not all patients identified as MCI will later develop dementia (Ganguli, Dodge et al., 2004; Larrieu et al., 2002; Wolf et al., 1998) clinicians are also interested to know the characteristics of those considered at high risk to convert. From a statistical point of view, one way to examine the predictive validity of a test is to construct Receiver Operating Characteristic (ROC) curves. A ROC curve is a graphical representation of the true positive rate against the false positive rate for the different possible cutpoints of a diagnostic test. It allows establishment of the most appropriate threshold for a test, based on how well it classifies subjects into the relevant groups (Benson et al., 2005). Several indices can be calculated from the ROC curves: (a) sensitivity, i.e. the probability that a patient will be correctly identified by the test as having MCI or as «true positive»; (b) specificity, i.e. the probability that a patient who does not have MCI will be accurately classified by the test as «true negative»; (c) positive predictive value (PPV), i.e. the probability that a patient has MCI given a «positive» test result; and (d) negative predictive value (NPV), i.e. the probability that a patient does not have MCI given a «negative» test result (Warner, 2004). The PPV and NPV represent an estimate of the probability that a given screening result is an accurate classification for a given individual, which is of particular interest for the patient (Kobak, Mundt, and Katzelnick, 2000). The area under the ROC curves (AUC) is another statistic that can also be used as a measure of efficacy of the test. A screening measure that is no better than chance will obtain an AUC = 0.50. If the discrimination is optimal, the AUC will equal 1.0 (Derogatis and Lynn, 2000). The optimal cutoff is chosen by maximizing the sensitivity (identifying all true cases), while not compromising the specificity (excluding all true non cases) of a test (Warner, 2004). The risk associated with a false diagnosis (either positive or negative) must also be considered. For example, it is well known that MCI patients present a high risk to later develop dementia, and that available treatments are more effective when administered as soon as possible. On the other hand, a certain proportion of MCI patients will remain stable, if not reverse to normal, and in these situations, the pharmacological treatments may induce undesirable side-effects. Given the current knowledge on MCI and dementia, the sensitivity and specificity of a diagnostic test should be kept equal.

In clinical practice, sensitivity and specificity may have a limited value (Meiran, Stuss, Guzman, Lafleche, and Willmer, 1996; Warner, 2004). A more useful approach is to use Likelihood Ratios (LR) which assesses the value of a diagnostic test (Warner, 2004). The LR is the likelihood that a given test result would be expected in a patient with the target disorder (LR^+) compared to the likelihood that that same result would be expected in a patient without the target disorder (LR^-). Because they are «ratios», they do not vary in different populations or settings; they are thus independent of disease prevalence. Therefore, they allow for a quantification of the probability of disease in any individual. These indexes are calculated using formulas involving the sensitivity and specificity values.

Formulas:

LR^+ = sensitivity / (1- specificity) and LR^- = (1-sensitivity / specificity).

LR^+ represents the change in odds favoring disease given a «positive» test result. LR^- expresses the change in odds favoring disease given a «negative» test result. The general interpretation guidelines indicate that a likelihood ratio (LR) greater than 1 indicates that the test result is associated with the presence of the disease, whereas a LR less than 1 indicates that the test result is associated with the absence of the disease. Likelihood ratios above 10 and below 0.1 are considered to provide strong evidence to rule in or rule out diagnoses respectively in most circumstances (Jaeschke, Guyatt, and Lijmer, 2002).

From a methodological point of view, researchers could try to establish the capacity of a given screening test to detect individuals with MCI by using a cross-sectional design, i.e. by comparing performances between healthy elderly people and patients responding to the criteria of MCI. A poorer performance of patients with MCI compared with that of healthy elderly on the neuropsychological test would then suggest the presence of cognitive changes characteristic of the preclinical stages of AD (Collie and Maruff, 2000). Other studies may attempt to differentiate amongst a large cohort of non-demented elderly individuals, with MCI or not, those who will and those who will not develop dementia by using a longitudinal research design. The comparison between the baseline performance of the patients that evolve to AD (converters) and the baseline performance of those who remain cognitively healthy (non-converters) then serves to infer the characteristics of the prodromal phase of the disease (Collie and Maruff, 2000). Since there is still no strong objective «gold standard» inherent to the concept of MCI, its validity as a prodrome of AD is better demonstrated by the presence of follow-up data which allow to eventually confirm the development of dementia (Petersen and O'Brien, 2006; Xu, Meyer, Thornby, Chowdhury, and Quach, 2002). Consequently, the inferences from longitudinal studies are considered to be the most robust evidence.

The goal of this chapter is to critically and qualitatively review the psychometric qualities of some of the most popular cognitive screening tests in North America and Europe, in terms of their capacity to properly detect MCI as a prodromal dementia state, especially in regards to Alzheimer's disease. The following cognitive screening instruments will thus be studied: (a) the Mini-Mental State Examination or MMSE (Folstein, Folstein, and McHugh, 1975), which is the most world-wide used brief mental status test (Chetelat et al., 2005); (b) the Cambridge Examination for Mental Disorders for the Elderly – Cognition or CAMCOG (Roth et al., 1986), which is a very popular screening test, especially in Europe (Visser, Verhey, Jolles, and Jonker, 2002); (c) the Alzheimer's Disease Assessment Scale – Cognition or ADAS-Cog (Rosen, Mohs, and Davis, 1984), which is one of the mandatory outcome measures required by the Food and Drug Administration (FDA) in the USA for the cognition-enhancer drug trials; and (d) the Mattis Dementia Rating Scale or MDRS (Coblentz et al., 1973; Mattis, 1976), which is an instrument largely used both in clinical and research settings throughout the world (Lucas et al., 1998).

METHOD

MEDLINE, PsycInfo and Current Content databases were searched using the following key terms: «Mini-Mental State Examination», «Alzheimer's Disease Assessment Scale – Cognition», «Cambridge Examination for Mental Disorders for the Elderly – Cognition», «Mattis Dementia Rating Scale», «validity», «sensitivity», «specificity», and «Mild Cognitive

Impairment». English-language, peer-reviewed articles published between 1975 and 2006 were included. Studies were included in the review only if their goal was to properly identify individuals with MCI (criterion validity). Cross-sectional studies assessing cognition without diagnostic and/or control group comparisons, and single and multiple single-case design studies were excluded.

For the purpose of this review, all studies were grouped into three specific categories according to the robustness of the experimental design: (a) Class A: Retrospective or prospective studies that specifically aimed to assess the sensitivity and specificity values of the screening test to detect the MCI using a longitudinal research design; (b) Class B: Cross-sectional controlled studies that specifically aimed to assess the sensitivity and specificity of the screening test to detect MCI and (c) Class C: Cross-sectional controlled studies comparing the performances of the MCI, other diagnostic groups and/or healthy controls on screening tests or prospective longitudinal studies comparing the baseline performances on screening tests of MCI patients who converted and those who did not convert to dementia over time. When the likelihood ratios (LR) were not mentioned by the authors, they were computed provided that sufficient information was available in the article (see Tables 1, 2, 3 and 5).

RESULTS

Mini-Mental State Examination

Brief Description of the Instrument

The most widely used screening test is, undoubtedly, the Mini-Mental State Examination or MMSE (Folstein et al., 1975). Its popularity might be explained by its short administration time (between 5 and 10 minutes) and its easy use and scoring (Lezak, Howieson, and Loring, 2004; Strauss, Sherman, and Spreen, 2006). The MMSE is composed of 30 items assessing orientation to time and space, episodic memory (three-words registration and recall), attention, calculation, language (naming, sentence repetition and reading, three-step command execution, writing) and construction praxis (copy of overlapping pentagons). However, there is no measure of executive function. The global score of the MMSE ranges from 0 to 30. The MMSE has been found to be sensitive to age and education level (Nelson, Fogel, and Faust, 1986; Stuss, Meiran, Guzman, Lafleche, and Willmer, 1996). Therefore, population-based norms for age and education level have been developed for individuals aged from 18 to greater than 85 years old, with no education to having a Bachelor's degree or higher education (Crum, Anthony, Bassett, and Folstein, 1993).

Although the MMSE was first conceived to differentiate neurological and psychiatric patients (Folstein et al., 1975), it is frequently used for the screening of dementia amongst elderly population (McDowell, Kristjansson, Hill, and Hebert, 1997; Simard, 1998; Simard and van Reekum, 1999). Several studies show that the MMSE may help in the identification of patients with mild to severe dementia (Folstein et al., 1975; Jackson and Ramsdell, 1988), and can provide some differential information on several etiologies of dementia (Jean, Simard, Van Reekum, and Clarke, 2005; Spreen and Strauss, 1998). The MMSE has been criticized for its ceiling and floor effects in regards to, respectively, the detection of early cognitive signs of dementia, and the assessment of cognitive impairment in severe dementia (Nelson et al., 1986; Simard, 1998; Simard and van Reekum, 1999).

Review of the Studies Assessing the Criterion Validity of the MMSE for the Detection of MCI

Class A Studies

Six studies were found that specifically aimed to assess the criterion validity of the MMSE alone, in combination or against other tests, in detecting MCI (see Table 1). Three of these studies used a longitudinal research design and were thus included in Class A (Isella et al., 2006; Lehrner et al., 2005; Tang-Wai et al., 2003). Not surprisingly, the mean follow-up period for the two prospective studies was shorter (1.9 and 2 years) than for the retrospective study (5.6 years). The participants were mostly recruited from memory clinic settings except for the study of Tang-Wai et al. (2003) which also included subjects from the community.

Isella et al. (2006) contrasted the discriminative and predictive power of the Informant Questionnaire on Cognitive Decline in the Elderly (IQCODE) (Jorm and Korten, 1988) with that of the MMSE and a verbal episodic memory measure, the Rey Auditory Verbal Learning Test (RAVLT) (Rey, 1958), in 45 MCI patients, 30 subjects with various types of dementia (57% of AD) and 55 healthy controls (HC). The MCI patients were classified according to the nosology of Petersen (2001). However, 20% of them were suspected to have a subcortical vascular cognitive impairment. The clinician who made the diagnoses was not blind to the MMSE scores at baseline and follow-up evaluations. This situation may have induced a circularity bias. The MCI patients registered significantly lower MMSE baseline scores than HC (d = 1.46). However, the MMSE scores did not differ between the MCI patients who converted (n = 24) and those who did not convert (n = 21) to dementia (d = 0.61) (Isella et al., 2006). The average follow-up period was 1.4 years for converters and 2.9 years for non-converters. The accuracy of the MMSE as a screening instrument for MCI was calculated using a ROC analysis.

The best cutoff was 28-29 for a fair sensitivity value of 82% and specificity of 73%, which was very close to the values obtained by the IQCODE. The AUC for the MMSE was 0.84 (Isella et al., 2006). Unfortunately, the authors did not examine the efficacy of the MMSE in predicting the transition from MCI to dementia as they did for the other instruments. The principal limitations of this study were the short follow-up period, the small sample size and the heterogeneity of the MCI sample. Since different cognitive presentations of MCI could be indicators of various neurodegenerative diseases, the statistical treatment of all types of MCI combined limits the conclusions that can be drawn from these results.

Table 1. Results of the Studies Assessing the Criterion Validity of the MMSE for the detection of MCI

Authors (year)	SAMPLES	RESULTS FROM ROC analyses					OTHER RESULTS	EFFECT SIZE (*d*) (Total score)	
		Research DeSIGN (mean follow-up delay)	Cutoff Sensitivity / Specificity	PPV / NPV (%)	AUC (95% CI)	LR $^{+}$/ LR -		1	2
Class A studies									
Isella *et al.* (2006)	55 HC 27 A-MCI, 10 M-MCI, 8 S-MCI 17 AD, 5 FTD, 2 VaD, 3 mixed and 3 NS dementia	Prospective Longitudinal (min. = 2 years)	Cutoff = 28-29: 82% / 73%	71% / 83%	0.84 (.73 - .92)	3.03 / 0.25	- Overall accuracy = 77% - BL: dementia < MCI < HC on MMSE* Tot - Convert = nonConvert on BL- MMSE* score	1.46	0.61
Lehrner *et al.* (2005)	Norms from 263 HC (age range: 18-91 years) 114 A-MCI	Prospective Longitudinal (1.8 ± 0.7 years)	Cutoff = 27: 83% / 68%	25% / 97%	0.84 (.74 - .93)	2.59 / 0.25	- Overall prediction = 71% - BL: A-MCI < HC on MMSE Tot - Convert < nonConvert on BL MMSE Tot	vs A-MCI: 1.17	1.33
Tang-Wai *et al.* (2003)	788 stable HC 129 prevalent MCI 235 very mild AD (CDR= 0.5) 54 incident MCI or 21 AD	Retrospective Longitudinal (5.6 ± 3.1 years)	Cutoff = 24: N/R Cutoff = 29: 82% / 48%	N/R	0.75 (.70 - .80)	0.30 / 0.35	- Prevalent MCI < HC on MMSE* Tot and Orientation / Delayed recall items - HC = incident MCI / AD on BL MMSE Tot	1.00	0.13[3]
Class A studies									
Benson *et al.* (2005)	25 HC 26 MCI (CDR= 0.5) 10 mild AD (CDR= 1.0) 25 Dep patients	Cross-sectional controlled	Cutoff ≤ 27: 57% / 72%	69% / 88%	0.79	2.04 / 0.60	- MCI < HC only on MMSE Tot - MCI = Dep patients on MMSE Tot	5.94	
Li *et al.* (2006)	88 HC 37 MCI (CDR= 0.5) 19 mild or moderate AD (CDR= 1 or 2)	Cross-sectional controlled	Cutoff ≤ 26: 65% / 57% Cutoff ≤ 27: 81% / 48%	N/R	0.68	1.50 / 0.39	FN rate: Cut-off ≤ 26: 35%; Cut-off ≤ 27: 19% FP. rate: Cut-off ≤ 26: 43%; Cut-off ≤ 27: 52%	0.61	

Table 1. Results of the Studies Assessing the Criterion Validity of the MMSE for the detection of MCI (Continued)

Authors (year)	SAMPLES	RESULTS FROM ROC analyses					OTHER RESULTS	EFFECT SIZE (*d*) (Total score)	
		Research DeSIGN (mean follow-up delay)	Cutoff Sensitivity / Specificity	PPV / NPV (%)	AUC (95% CI)	LR $^+$ / LR -		1	2
Ravaglia *et al.* (2006)	55 HC 38 A-MCI (CDR= 0.5) 18 S-MCI (CDR= 0.5) 57 M-MCI (CDR= 0.5) 22 very mild AD (CDR= 0.5)	Cross-sectional controlled	Cutoff = 24: To A-MCI, 29% / 87% To S-MCI, 44% / 87% To M-MCI, 49% / 87%	N/R	N/R	2.23 / 0.82	- A-MCI and S-MCI = HC on MMSE* Tot - M-MCI < HC on MMSE* Tot	vs A-MCI: 0.32 vs S-MCI: 0.48 vs M-MCI: 0.88	
Class C studies									
Wang & Zhou (2002)	20 HC 20 MCI	Cross-sectional controlled	N/R	N/R	N/R	N/R	- MCI = HC on MMSE* Tot	0.47	
Boeve *et al.* (2003)	56 HC 13 A-MCI 42 degenerative dementia	Cross-sectional controlled	N/R	N/R	N/R	N/R	- A-MCI = HC on MMSE Tot	0.56	
Grundman *et al.* (2004)	107 HC 769 A-MCI (CDR= 0.5) 122 very mild AD (CDR= 0.5) 183 mild AD (CDR= 1.0)	Cross-sectional controlled	N/R	N/R	N/R	N/R	- A-MCI < HC on MMSE* Tot	1.13	
Lam *et al.* (2005)	78 HC (CDR= 0) 76 QD patients (CDR= 0.5)	Cross-sectional controlled	N/R	N/R	N/R	N/R	- QD < HC on MMSE Tot - MMSE isn't a significant predictor of group membership	1.32	
Pyo *et al.* (2006)	843 HC 135 MCI (CDR= 0.5) 30 AD (CDR= 0.5) 125 AD (CDR= 1)	Cross-sectional controlled	N/R	N/R	N/R	N/R	- MCI < HC on MMSE* Tot	1.33	
Perneczky *et al.* (2006)	30 HC 45 MCI (CDR= 0.5)	Cross-sectional controlled	N/R	N/R	N/R	N/R	- MCI < HC on MMSE* Tot	2.25	

Table 1. Results of the Studies Assessing the Criterion Validity of the MMSE for the detection of MCI (Continued)

Authors (year)	SAMPLES	RESULTS FROM ROC analyses					OTHER RESULTS	EFFECT SIZE (*d*) (Total score)	
		Research DeSIGN (mean follow-up delay)	Cutoff Sensitivity / Specificity	PPV / NPV (%)	AUC (95% CI)	LR $^{+}$/ LR -		1	2
Tabert *et al.* (2006)	83 HC 21 A-MCI 20 S-MCI 87 M-MCI 20 cognitively impaired >1.5 SD cutoff threshold	Prospective Longitudinal (3.8 years ± 2.1)	N/R	N/R	N/R	NR/	- BL: MCI < HC on MMSE* Tot - Follow-up 1 year: 30 Convert vs 109 nonConvert - Follow-up 3 years: 35 Convert vs 80 nonConvert - Convert (1 and 3 years) < nonConvert on BL MMSE* Tot	1.5	1 year: 0.93 3 years: 0.98
van der Flier *et al.* (2005)	28 HC 20 M-Com subjects 17 MCI	Prospective Longitudinal (1.8 years)	N/R	N/R	N/R	N/R	- BL: mCom < HC on MMSE* Tot - Follow-up: 10 Convert vs 23 nonConvert - Convert < nonConvert on BL MMSE* Tot	1.0	2.00
Tian *et al.* (2003)	135 QD patients (CDR= 0.5)	Prospective Longitudinal (2.0 ± 1.6 years)	N/R	N/R	N/R	N/R	- Follow-up : 37 Convert vs 92 nonConvert - Convert < nonConvert on BL: MMSE* Tot - MMSE* Tot isn't a significant predictor of final diagnosis of dementia		0.69
Visser *et al.* (2001)	MCI patients[4] 25 very mild AD	Prospective Longitudinal (5 years)	N/R	N/R	N/R	N/R	- Follow-up : 23 Convert vs 44 nonConvert - Convert < nonConvert on BL MMSE* Tot score - MMSE* Tot isn't a significant predictor of final diagnosis of dementia		0.97

Table 1. Results of the Studies Assessing the Criterion Validity of the MMSE for the detection of MCI (Continued)

Authors (year)	SAMPLES	RESULTS FROM ROC analyses: Research DeSIGN (mean follow-up delay)	Cutoff Sensitivity / Specificity	PPV / NPV (%)	AUC (95% CI)	LR +/ LR -	OTHER RESULTS	EFFECT SIZE (*d*) (Total score) 1	2
Visser *et al.* (2002)	63 patients with «minimal dementia»	Prospective Longitudinal (2.3 ± 0.8 years)	N/R	N/R	N/R	N/R	- Follow-up: 24 Convert vs 10 nonConvert - Convert = nonConvert on BL MMSE* Tot - MMSE* Tot isn't a significant predictor of final diagnosis of dementia		- 0.23
Griffith *et al.* (2006)	49 HC 49 A-MCI (CDR= 0.5)	Prospective Longitudinal (1.1 year)	N/R	N/R	N/R	N/R	- BL: A-MCI = HC on MMSE Tot - Follow-up: 13 Convert vs 36 nonConvert - Convert = nonConvert on BL MMSE	0.49	0.14

Note. Class A: Longitudinal (retrospective or prospective) studies that specifically aimed to assess the sensitivity and specificity values of the MMSE to detect the MCI; Class B: Cross-sectional controlled studies that specifically aimed to assess the sensitivity and specificity of the MMSE to detect the MCI; Class C: Cross-sectional controlled studies comparing the performances of the MCI, other diagnostic groups and/or healthy controls on the MMSE or prospective longitudinal studies comparing the baseline performances on the MMSE of MCI who converted and those who did not convert to dementia over time.

PPV = Positive predictive value; NPV = Negative predictive value; AUC = Area under ROC curve; BL= baseline; LR^+ / LR^- = Positive / Negative Likelihood ratios; FN = False negative; FP= False positive; NS = Not specified; N/R = Not reported

S-MCI = Single-non-memory domain MCI; A-MCI = Amnesic MCI; M-MCI = Multiple-domain MCI; M-Com = subjective Memory Complaints;

HC = Healthy controls; AD = Alzheimer disease; VaD = Vascular dementia; FTD = Fronto-temporal dementia, QD = Questionable dementia; Dep = Depression

Convert = MCI converters to dementia; nonConvert = MCI non-converters to dementia

CDR = Clinical Dementia Rating scale score; MMSE Tot = Mini-Mental State Examination total score;

* MMSE Total score is part of the selection procedure for MCI or dementia or is available for diagnosis at baseline (circularity bias)

[1] HC vs prevalent MCI [2] Convert vs Non convert [3] Stable HC vs incident MCI or AD [4] Number of MCI at the entry of the study is not reported

In an attempt to assess the predictive value of several neuropsychological tests, Lehrner et al. (2005) followed 114 amnesic MCI (A-MCI) for an average of 1.9 years. At the second evaluation, 13.1% of them were diagnosed as having AD, with an annual conversion rate of 6.5%. After correction for multiplicity, the baseline MMSE score was significantly different between healthy controls (HC) and A-MCI ($d = 1.17$), as well as between converters to AD ($n = 12$) and non-converters ($n = 93$) ($d = 1.33$) (Lehrner et al., 2005). The sensitivity / specificity estimates were calculated for a cutoff score of 27. The values of these particular indices as well as those of the AUC were very similar to the results obtained by Isella et al. (2006). Interestingly, the authors addressed the question whether grouping the subjects into A-MCI and HC groups using similar criteria to Peterson et al. (1999) can accurately predict the future development of dementia. The analyses revealed sensitivity / specificity estimates of respectively 83% and 68%, PPV / NPV values of 25% and 97% respectively, and an overall correct prediction percentage of 71% (Lehrner et al., 2005). These last results added to the construct validity of the A-MCI concept while suggesting that this grouping strategy could fail to detect several individuals who will become demented. Generalization of this finding is limited by the small sample size which restricted the number of incident dementia cases (Lehrner et al., 2005).

The last class A study was conducted by Tang-Wai et al. (2003) who retrospectively compared the MMSE and the Short Test of Mental Status (STMS) (Kokmen, Naessens, and Offord, 1987) baseline scores regarding their efficacy to detect future MCI patients. The authors grouped the subjects according to their diagnostic status at follow-up using the following terms: stable normal (normal cognition at baseline and follow-up), prevalent (MCI at baseline and follow-up) and incident MCI (MCI only at follow-up), prevalent and incident AD. They then performed analyses for which they grouped subjects according to their baseline and follow-up Clinical Dementia Rating scale (CDR) (Morris, 1993) scores (Tang-Wai et al., 2003). Significant differences at baseline between the HC and prevalent MCI on the scores of Orientation and Delayed recall subtests and total score of the MMSE ($d = 1.0$) were found. However, the MMSE Total score and the scores of the subtests did not-identify individuals with normal cognition at baseline who converted to MCI or AD during the follow-up period ($d = 0.13$) (Tang-Wai et al., 2003). A cutoff score of 29 on the MMSE at baseline had 82% sensitivity but only 48% specificity to later detect prevalent MCI. ROC analyses seemed to have been calculated using the usual cutoff score of 24 for dementia, but the authors did not report the results of this analysis; they instead commented them. They apparently found very poor sensitivity and high specificity for the MMSE to detect MCI using this low cutoff score, which is consistent with the results of Tombaugh and McIntyre (1992). In a comprehensive review of evidence on MMSE, they demonstrated that a cutoff of 23/24 showed high sensitivity to moderate to severe cognitive impairment, but less sensitivity to milder impairment (Tombaugh and McIntyre, 1992). This strongly suggests that if using the usual cutoff score of 24 for dementia, one could certainly miss individuals at a preclinical state. The study conducted by Tang-Wai et al. had some limitations. The HC subjects were slightly younger than the prevalent MCI patients which could account for the differences found between the two groups. The clinicians who diagnosed the patients were not blind to the MMSE and STMS scores; there was therefore a risk for circularity bias. Although the authors addressed the circularity issue by grouping patients per their CDR scores (at baseline and follow-up), and per their diagnosis at follow-up, the strategies used are of limited value considering that both the MMSE and STMS were performed at the two evaluation points i.e. at baseline and follow-up.

Class B Studies

In their cross-sectional controlled study, Benson, Slavin, Tran, Petrella and Doraiswamy (2005) found that the total MMSE score was able to distinguish the 25 HC from 26 MCI patients, even when age, sex and education were considered in the analyses of covariance. However, no significant differences on the individual items scores emerged. The result of the effect size calculation was 5.94, but the difference between the mean scores obtained by the two groups was small (1.9). The sensitivity of the optimal cutoff score (27) for MCI was only of 57%. Moreover, the performance of the MCI patients was comparable to the performance of 25 depressive patients on the overall MMSE score (Benson et al., 2005).

A higher sensitivity value was obtained with Chinese participants (Li, Ng, Kua, and Ko, 2006) using the same cutoff score as that of Benson et al. (2005), but at the cost of a higher false positive rate than when a cutoff score of 26 was used (see Table 1). In addition, this group of researchers found that, when the MMSE was compared to other neuropsychological tests such as the subtests Logical Memory I and II from the Wechsler Memory Scale (WMS), the MMSE had the weakest power to distinguish HC from the MCI individuals (AUC = 0.68). The authors did not mention which version of the WMS they used nor the reference of the test. They concluded that the performance on the MMSE was not a good predictor of group membership (Li et al., 2006). This conclusion is supported by a small effect size (below 1.0), as can be seen in Table 1.

The values obtained by Ravaglia et al. (2005) further confirmed that the total MMSE score was not a good indicator of group membership (effect size below 1.0). A cutoff score of 24 on the MMSE was used to compare the performance of 55 HC and 113 MCI participants attending a University memory clinic. Only the M-MCI group could be differentiated from the HC on this basis ($d = 0.88$). However, the inclusion of controls presenting with subjective memory complaints, but judged cognitively and functionally intact according to a geriatric evaluation and neuropsychological testing (results of their tests were $\geq$ - 1.5 SD per the reference norms), could have reduced the differences between the two groups (Ravaglia et al., 2005).

The principal limitations of the three class B studies were the small sample size and the absence of longitudinal data. Taken together, their results suggest that the MMSE is not a sensitive measure to detect MCI. In addition, the MMSE might not be appropriate to differentially diagnose cognitive impairment caused by depression versus that inherent to MCI.

Class C Studies

Fourteen studies were found to belong to Class C (see Table 1). One of them was rejected (Lee et al., 2006) because of a lack of information in the method and result sections that prevented an appropriate appraisal of their results. Another study was rejected because it was a multiple single-case research design (Hodges, Erzinclioglu, and Patterson, 2006). The remaining 12 studies did not specifically aim to evaluate sensitivity and specificity of the MMSE, and all but two studies (Boeve et al., 2003; Lam, Lui, Chiu, and Chan, 2006) considered the total score of the MMSE as one of the selection criteria for MCI or dementia. A circularity bias is thus induced by this procedure.

Six studies used a cross-sectional controlled research design (Boeve et al., 2003; Grundman et al., 2004; Lam et al., 2006; Perneczky, Pohl, Sorg, Hartmann, Komossa et al., 2006; Pyo, Elble, Ala, and Markwell, 2006; Wang and Zhou, 2002), and six studies used a prospective longitudinal research design (Grundman et al., 2004; Lam, Lui, Chiu, and Chan, 2005; Pyo et al., 2006; Tabert et al., 2006; Visser, Verhey, Ponds, and Jolles, 2001). Two of the cross-sectional studies did not find any significant difference between the total MMSE score obtained by the MCI versus that of the HC participants (Boeve et al., 2003; Wang and Zhou, 2002).Wang and Zhou (2002) used the MMSE for diagnostic purpose in a study evaluating retrieval and encoding capacities in patients with MCI and normal aging. They did not find any significant difference between the MCI patients (n = 20; mean = 26.2 ± 1.5) and the HC (n = 20; mean = 25.5 ± 1.5) on the MMSE (d = 0.47). The small sample size, inducing poor statistical power, could be responsible for this non-significant result. Boeve et al. (2003) also did not find significant differences between the total MMSE scores of 56 HC (mean = 27.9 ± 2.3) and 13 A-MCI (mean = 26.8 ± 1.6) recruited among the oldest old (the mean age of this particular sample was 94.1 ± 2.6 years old).

Four other cross-sectional studies demonstrated that the MMSE was able to detect MCI in individuals living in the community (Grundman et al., 2004; Lam et al., 2005; 2006; Pyo et al., 2006), and attending a university-based clinic on cognition (Perneczky, Pohl, Sorg, Hartmann, Komossa et al., 2006). The mean MMSE scores registered by the MCI patients in these studies versus those registered by the HC ranged respectively from 27.3 ± 1.9 to 29.1 ± 1.3, from 23.4 ± 4.3 to 27.7 ± 2.1, from 26.4 ± 2.6 to 28.9± 1.2 and from 26.9 ± 1.4 to 29.3 ± 0.7. The effect sizes varied from 1.13 (Grundman et al., 2004) to 2.25 (Perneczky, Pohl, Sorg, Hartmann, Komossa et al., 2006). The highest effect size was obtained with patients recruited in a clinical setting (Perneczky, Pohl, Sorg, Hartmann, Komossa et al., 2006), and who were thus more likely to present a more advanced cognitive decline than MCI participants recruited from the community (Lehrner et al., 2005).

Six Class C studies were prospectively conceived and followed their participants for periods from 1.8 (van der Flier et al., 2005) to 5 years (Visser et al., 2001). In order to evaluate conversion rates to AD in subtypes of MCI, and to identify neuropsychological measures most predictive of the time to conversion, Tabert et al. (2006) compared performances of 148 MCI patients of different subtypes and 63 group-matched controls. The total MMSE score was used as selection criteria for the MCI (MMSE ≥ 22) and the HC (MMSE ≥ 27) groups, thus leading to a significant difference between these two groups at baseline (d = 1.2). MCI patients who later developed AD after 1 (n = 30) and 3 (n = 35) years of follow-up initially performed worse on MMSE than the MCI patients who remained stable (Tabert et al., 2006). Restricting the sample to a three year follow-up, 50% of the M-MCI (multiple domains plus amnesia) patients against 10% of pure amnesic patients converted to AD. This finding confirmed the higher risk of conversion for this subtype observed in other studies (Bozoki, Giordani, Heidebrink, Berent, and Foster, 2001). Van der Flier et al. (2005) investigated whether MRI-based volumes could predict the progression of cognitive decline. They reported that patients with MCI had lower scores (mean = 26 ± 2) on the MMSE than HC (mean = 28 ± 2) (d = 1.0) and subjects with only memory complaints (mean = 29 ± 1) at baseline. In addition, one patient with subjective memory complaints and nine MCI patients who converted to probable AD during follow-up had weaker performances at baseline on the MMSE than participants who did not develop dementia (d = 2.0) (van der Flier et al., 2005).

The relative efficacy of the MMSE to distinguish patients responding to the criteria for «questionable dementia» (QD) who converted versus those who did not convert to dementia was also demonstrated by Tian, Bucks, Haworth and Wilcock (2003). QD is defined by a Clinical Dementia Rating (CDR) of 0.5 (Hughes, Berg, Danziger, Coben, and Martin, 1982). The QD patients who declined cognitively were older (mean age = 73.2 ± 8.5) at entry in the study than those who did not decline (mean age = 68.7 ± 10.2) (Tian, Bucks, Haworth, and Wilcock, 2003). The effect size between both group performances was small (d = 0.69), and the MMSE total score was not a consistent predictor of future development of dementia. It was a significant predictor in only one out of six Cox regression models while age was moderately and positively associated with increased risk of converting to dementia (Tian et al., 2003). In the same way, Visser et al. (2001) demonstrated that the MMSE was not able to accurately predict the final diagnosis of dementia after a 5-year follow-up period. Nevertheless, the MMSE total score was slightly lower in MCI converters to dementia than in non-progressive MCI patients (d = 0.97).

Finally, two groups of authors did not find any significant difference on baseline total MMSE score between MCI converters and non-converters after approximately one year (Griffith et al., 2006) and two years of follow-up (Visser, Verhey, Hofman, Scheltens, and Jolles, 2002). The small number of participants at study entry (respectively 49 and 63 patients) combined with the short follow-up period might have greatly reduced the possibility of finding newly diagnosed dementia patients in their sample (respectively 13 and 24 converters). Consequently, the absence of difference could be explained, in part, by a lack of statistical power.

Discussion of the MMSE Results

Taken together, the reviewed evidence did not provide consistent data in favor of the use of the MMSE for the detection of MCI. The longitudinal studies demonstrated that good sensitivity values were always obtained at the cost of lower specificity and the reverse is true. The PPV / NPV indices also suggested that the MMSE was better in identifying the individuals free of MCI who will not progress to dementia in future years (NPV range: 83% to 97%). Xu et al. (2002) affirmed that PPV of the MMSE should increase with longer follow-up. This was not confirmed by the studies reviewed. However, the magnitude of the effect increases with decreasing time between cognitive assessment and diagnosis, which is congruent with patterns noted by other authors (Backman, Jones, Berger, Laukka, and Small, 2004). On the other hand, it has been proposed that, because of its poor sensitivity values in community-dwelling people, the MMSE should be reserved to specific populations, like those attending memory clinics or residing in assisted facilities, where the highest rates of dementia are expected (Tangalos et al., 1996). However, our findings did not show that the efficacy of the MMSE in differentiating MCI patients and HC was better in clinical settings than in the community. Indeed, the effect size varied from 0.32 to 2.25 in memory clinics, and from 1.32 to 5.94 in population-based studies. Moreover, the cross-sectional research design could not totally account for these findings, since the effect size was no better in prospective longitudinal studies. Nevertheless, when comparing the positive likelihood ratio (LR^+) values, the average probability of the presence of MCI given a particular MMSE cutoff score was higher in clinical (mean LR^+ = 2.86) than in community settings (mean LR^+ = 1.28). Thus, from a clinical point of view, the MMSE gives only little information for ruling in or out the diagnosis of MCI.

Several factors may account for the poor performances of the MMSE, and many of these factors have been mentioned in the literature. First, the MMSE total score is inversely proportional to age (Crum et al., 1993; Tombaugh, McDowell, Kristjansson, and Hubley, 1996). Although Crum et al. (1993) provided norms according to age and educational level, none of the reviewed studies herein presented utilized these norms to correct the MMSE scores of their participants. Poor educational level could lead to a false diagnosis of cognitive impairment while superior education could hinder the presence of MCI (Spreen and Strauss, 1998). Nevertheless, educational levels seemed not to account entirely for the inconsistent sensitivity of the MMSE. For example, in the reviewed studies providing sensitivity / specificity values, the false positive rate ([1-specificity] x 100) using a cutoff of 29 was 52% amongst people who completed an average of 13 years of schooling (Tang-Wai et al., 2003), and 27% amongst people who completed only 7 years of schooling (Isella et al., 2006).

Other possible explanatory factors to be mentioned are related to the cognitive processes known to be affected in MCI and early AD, and that are not assessed by the MMSE. The different episodic memory processes (encoding, retention, retrieval and consolidation) aren't well evaluated by the MMSE (Simard and van Reekum, 1999), while various administration differences regarding the memory delay subsist (Fields, 1998; Milberg, 1996). Another problem with the administration of this instrument is the choice that clinicians have to administer either the item «spelling WORLD backwards» or the item «counting backwards, in units of seven, starting with 100». These two tasks do not have the same requirements in terms of attentional demands; the first task is less demanding than the second one. In addition, the MMSE over-assesses verbal abilities to the detriment of other cognitive functions, especially the executive functions (Fields, 1998; Spreen and Strauss, 1998; Strauss et al., 2006). However, if the current conception of MCI generally implies a memory decline, other variants of MCI involving impairments in a single or multiple cognitive domains are now recognized (Peterson and Morris, 2003). Recent research also demonstrated a heterogeneous cognitive presentation in about 14% of individuals with AD (Morris and Becker, 2004; Morris and James, 2004). The American Psychological Association (1998) published guidelines for the assessment of age-consistent memory decline and dementia. The task force pointed out the importance of using standardized neuropsychological tests to evaluate a range of cognitive functions including memory, attention, perceptual and motor skills, language, visuo-spatial skills, problem solving and executive functions (American Psychiatric Association, 1998). Consequently, an effective screening test should encompass the whole spectrum of cognitive functions that might be affected in preclinical and mild AD (Patterson et al., 2001).

CAMBRIDGE EXAMINATION FOR MENTAL DISORDERS FOR THE ELDERLY - COGNITION (CAMCOG)

Brief Description of the Instrument

The CAMCOG is the cognitive part of the Cambridge Examination for Mental Disorders for the Elderly (or CAMDEX) that was developed in the United Kingdom (Roth et al., 1986). It includes 14 of 19 items from the MMSE as well as 43 additional items. When used in clinical settings, the possible maximum score is 107. However when the CAMCOG is administered in the community, the possible maximum score is usually 106 because the subject cannot answer the question asking to recognize people such as doctors or nurses. The original version of the CAMCOG covers the cognitive domains of language, orientation, attention, memory, abstract thinking, calculation, perception and praxis. However, it does not assess executive functions.

The first results on the criterion validity of the CAMCOG were reported by Roth and al. (1986). Their sample included 49 demented patients with moderate to severe impairment (mean MMSE score = 13.4, range 1-25). Examination of the distribution of scores showed the optimal cutoff to be 79/80, yielding to a sensitivity of 92% and a specificity of 96% (Roth et al., 1986). It was later demonstrated that age and education strongly affect the total score on the CAMCOG (Huppert et al., 1996; Lindeboom, Ter Horst, Hooyer, Dinkgreve, and Jonker, 1993). This finding prompted the development of normative data according to these two demographic variables (Lolk, Nielsen, Andersen, Andersen, and Kragh-Sorensen, 2000; Williams, Huppert, Matthews, and Nickson, 2003). Sex and education were also shown to have significant independent effects on CAMCOG total score and on many of the CAMCOG subscales (Huppert et al., 1996).

The CAMDEX uses the term «minimal dementia» to describe patients wild mild cognitive impairment at high risk for dementia (Roth et al., 1986). The diagnosis of minimal dementia is made according to overall clinical impression when patients do not meet the stringent criteria for dementia (e.g. DSM-IV), and present with a limited and variable impairment in cognition such as difficulties with learning and recalling events, a tendency to misplace possessions, and minor errors in orientation (Roth et al., 1986). However, the optimal cutoff score for the detection of mild cognitive impairment using the CAMCOG remains unknown (Blessed, Black, Butler, and Kay, 1991).

Review of the Studies Assessing the Criterion Validity of the CAMCOG for the Detection of MCI

Only five studies provided data on the criterion validity of the CAMCOG in regards to the MCI population (see Table 2). Two Class A studies (Fountoulakis, Tsolakis, and Kazis, 2001; Huppert et al., 1996) were excluded because the participants with MCI were integrated into the dementia group, and the analyses were performed on this integrated group only. The remaining three studies met the Class C criteria. The MCI patients were gathered from a community-dwelling population enrolled in another larger study on mental health functioning

(Visser, Verhey, Jolles et al., 2002) or were referred for cognitive evaluation at a specialized clinic (van der Flier et al., 2005; Wang and Zhou, 2002).

Class C Studies

As part of the diagnostic session, Wang and Zhou (2002) administered a Chinese adapted version of the CAMCOG to 20 HC and 20 MCI participants. These subjects were comparable on education and age variables. Although the total scores of the MCI patients fell in the normal range (CAMCOG cutoff was 79-80), their total scores were significantly poorer than those of the HC group ($d = 0.50$). The MCI patients also performed poorly on four subscales, i.e. the *Orientation*, *Language*, *Memory* and *Praxis* subscales. The inferior performance on the *Memory* subtest was the most obvious ($d = 2.84$) (Wang and Zhou, 2002). This result was not surprising since the MCI patients were selected because of their isolated memory impairment, and also because the scores of the CAMCOG scale were made available to the clinician at the time of diagnosis. Consequently, a circularity bias might be responsible for this particular finding.

In order to investigate whether or not MRI-based volume measures could predict the progression of cognitive decline, van der Flier et al. (2005) followed 28 HC, 20 individuals with memory complaints, and 17 patients with MCI over a mean follow-up period of 1.8 years. The attrition rate was small, i.e. 9%. The general cognitive function, as assessed by the CAMCOG, was lower in the MCI than in the HC group at baseline ($d = 2.9$). The CAMCOG total score at baseline was also poorer in the MCI patients who developed dementia than in those who remained stable over time ($d = 2.40$) (van der Flier et al., 2005). The number of participants per groups was small, and few of them converted to dementia. It is possible that a higher proportion of participants would have shown a progression towards cognitive decline with a longer follow-up period.

Unlike the previous studies that used Petersen's criteria for the diagnosis of MCI, Visser et al. (2002) followed a cohort of 63 patients responding to the «minimal dementia» criteria (Roth et al., 1986) during an average of 2.3 years. Among these patients, 24 individuals declined and received a diagnosis of dementia, 10 patients remained stable whereas 11 reversed to normal (Visser, Verhey, Jolles et al., 2002). There was no difference at baseline between the CAMCOG total scores of the converters and non-converters. However, following a logistic regression analysis (backward method), age, the presence of APOE ϵ_4 and the baseline CAMCOG *Memory* subscale score were retained as predictors for dementia (Visser, Verhey, Jolles et al., 2002). The baseline CAMCOG *Memory* score was also retained as the only predictor for reversible minimal dementia. However, one should mention that the CAMCOG total score was not entered in the logistic regression analysis because there was multilinearity with other cognitive measures (e.g. MMSE). The authors recommended applying a cutoff score on the *Memory* subscale < 19 (if age > 75 years) to predict future development of dementia, and a cutoff score ≥ 19 (if age ≤ 78 years) to identify subjects with reversible dementia. Though appealing, these suggested cutoffs require cross-validation (Visser, Verhey, Jolles et al., 2002). This longitudinal study had however an important attrition rate (30%).

Table 2. Results of the Studies Assessing the Criterion Validity of the CAMCOG for the Detection of MCI

Authors (year)	SAMPLES	Research Device (mean follow-up delay)	RESULTS FROM ROC analyses			LR + / LR -	OTHER RESULTS	EFFECT SIZE (*d*) (Total score)	
			Cutoff Sensitivity / Specificity	PPV / NPV (%)	AUC (95% CI)			1	2
Class A studies									
Class B studies									
Class C studies									
Wang & Zhou (2002)	20 HC 20 MCI	Prospective Cross-sectional	N/R	N/R	N/R	N/R	- MCI < HC on CAMCOG* Tot and on Orientation, Language, Memory and Praxis subscales	0.50	
van der Flier *et al.* (2005)	28 HC 20 mCom subjects 17 MCI	Prospective Longitudinal (1.8 years)	N/R	N/R	N/R	N/R	- BL: MCI < mCom and HC on CAMCOG* Tot - Follow-up: 10 Convert vs 23 nonConvert - Convert < nonConvert on BL CAMCOG* Tot	2.90	2.40

Table 2. (Continued)

Authors (year)	SAMPLES	Research Device (mean follow-up delay)	RESULTS FROM ROC analyses Cutoff Sensitivity / Specificity	PPV / NPV (%)	AUC (95% CI)	LR^+ / LR^-	OTHER RESULTS	EFFECT SIZE (*d*) (Total score) 1	2
Visser *et al.* (2002)	63 patients with «minimal dementia»	Prospective Longitudinal (2.3 ± 0.8 years)	N/R	N/R	N/R	N/R	- Follow-up: 24 Convert vs 10 nonConvert - Convert = nonConvert on BL CAMCOG* Tot - Age > 75 years and BL CAMCOG-memory score < 19 are best predictors of final diagnosis of dementia		0.38

Note. Class A: Longitudinal (retrospective or prospective) studies that specifically aimed to assess the sensitivity and specificity values of the CAMCOG to detect the MCI; Class B: Cross-sectional controlled studies that specifically aimed to assess the sensitivity and specificity of the CAMCOG to detect the MCI; Class C: Cross-sectional controlled studies comparing the performances of the MCI, other diagnostic groups and/or healthy controls on the CAMCOG or prospective longitudinal studies comparing the baseline performances on the CAMCOG of MCI who converted and those who did not convert to dementia over time.

PPV = Positive predictive value; NPV = Negative predictive value; AUC = Area under ROC curve; BL = baseline; LR^+ / LR^- = Positive / Negative Likelihood ratios; N/R = Not reported; MCI = Mild Cognitive Impairment; HC = Healthy Controls; mCom: subjective Memory Complaints;

Convert = MCI converters to dementia; nonConvert = MCI non-converters to dementia; CAMCOG Tot: CAMCOG total score

* CAMCOG Total score is part of the selection criteria for MCI or dementia or score available for diagnosis at baseline (circularity bias)

Effect size[1] =HC vs prevalent MCI ; Effect size [2] =Convert vs Non convert

Discussion of the CAMCOG Results

The findings of Wang and Zhou (2002), van der Flier et al. (2005), and Visser et al. (2002) provided some support for the utilization of the CAMCOG in the detection of MCI patients who are at high risk to develop dementia of various etiologies. However, the results came from only three studies that were not specifically aimed to assess the sensitivity and specificity of the CAMCOG for the diagnosis of MCI. Consequently, it was not possible to calculate the LR. In addition, the small sample size and the short (if not absent) follow-up periods were strong limitations of these studies. Moreover, the participants in these studies completed an average of 8.6 years of schooling. The CAMCOG could thus be less efficacious to detect a preclinical state of dementia in individuals presenting with higher levels of education. The validity of the CAMCOG as a diagnostic tool for MCI will have to be further investigated in future research using a prospective longitudinal design, blinded diagnosis at baseline in regards to the CAMCOG scores, and greater sample size.

The Alzheimer's Disease Assessment Scale - Cognition (ADAS - Cog)

Brief Description of the Instrument

The ADAS (Rosen et al., 1984) includes two sections. The first part assesses the severity of behavioural and psychiatric dysfunctions found in AD (ADAS-non-Cog) and the second part, the severity of cognitive impairment (ADAS-Cog). The ADAS-Cog has a negative scoring system, i.e. the highest score represents the worst performance whereas the lowest score represents the best possible performance. The possible maximum (total) score is 69. The ADAS-Cog covers five general cognitive functions through 11 sections: (a) language (subjective observations on spontaneous speech, oral comprehension, and word-finding difficulty), commands execution and naming (objects and fingers); (b) ideational praxis (folding a sheet of paper and putting it in an envelop); (c) constructional praxis (copying geometric designs); (d) orientation, and (e) memory (10-word list learning and immediate recognition). The administration time of the ADAS-Cog varies between 20 to 45 minutes, and it can be administered to demented patients with several degrees of cognitive impairment (Zec et al., 1992).

However, some critic has been addressed to the ADAS-Cog. Like the MMSE, the ADAS-Cog under-evaluates the executive and posterior cognitive functions (Simard and van Reekum, 1999). In addition, it does not assess important aspects of cognition such as semantic memory, and the encoding and consolidation processes involved in episodic memory (Simard and van Reekum, 1999). While these functions are amongst the first altered in AD, it can greatly reduce the ADAS-Cog's capacity to identify people affected by the disease in the early stages, resulting in a higher rate of false negatives. In order to remedy this situation, researchers often add a five-minute-delayed recall to the usual memory task (Grundman et al., 2004; Pyo et al., 2006). Knowing how well or not the ADAS-Cog might be sensitive to MCI is important because despite its limitations, it is one of the most administered cognitive measures in drug trials for patients-in various levels of AD (Pyo et al., 2006).

Review of the Studies Assessing the Criterion Validity of the ADAS-Cog for the Detection of MCI

Only four studies provided data on the criterion validity of the ADAS-Cog in regards to the detection of MCI (see Table 3). Two of these studies corresponded to Class B's description (Perneczky, Pohl, Sorg, Hartmann, Komossa et al., 2006; Pyo et al., 2006), whereas two studies met the criteria of Class C (Grundman et al., 2004; Lam et al., 2006). They all used a cross-sectional controlled research design, and thus did not report any follow-up data. The MCI patients were recruited among community-dwelling individuals (Grundman et al., 2004; Lam et al., 2006; Pyo et al., 2006), or among those who sought, or were referred for cognitive evaluation at a specialized clinic (Perneczky, Pohl, Sorg, Hartmann, Komossa et al., 2006; Pyo et al., 2006).

Class B Studies

Pyo *et al.* (2006) investigated the usefulness of the ADAS-Cog for the diagnosis of MCI and the effects of demographic variables on performance. They recruited 843 HC who were population-based volunteers enrolled in another large study on aging, 135 MCI patients with a CDR score = 0.5 who were referred to a neurology clinic, 30 AD patients with a CDR score = 0.5, and 125 AD patients with a CDR score = 1.0. The HC were significantly more educated than the other groups (Pyo et al., 2006). The ADAS-Cog scores of the MCI group were significantly higher than the scores of the HC group on the total number of errors ($d = 1.74$), and on all the subtests. However, the authors reported that the MCI patients made the major part of the errors on the memory subtests, principally on *Word recall* and *Word recognition* (*Delayed Memory recall* score was not included in this analysis). The mean scores on non-memory subtests were in the range of only 0.10 to 0.87 (Pyo et al., 2006). The use of Conover's method to correct for multiple comparisons might be responsible for the results because this method exhibited a tendency to overestimate distinctness underlying populations and to falsely declare «different» populations being in fact identical (Rublìk, 2001).

Perneczky et al. (2006) tried to verify if cognitive testing using the ADAS-Cog and assessment of activities of daily living (ADL) using the Alzheimer's disease Cooperative Study scale for Activities of Daily Living (ADSC-MCI-ADL) (Galasko et al., 1997) were significant predictors of the diagnosis of MCI. Their sample was composed of 45 MCI and 30 age-matched controls. For the purposes of the study, Petersen's criteria for the diagnosis of MCI were modified in three ways: (a) subjective memory complaints were not required, (b) memory impairment may be absent if at least one other cognitive domains was significantly affected (at least 1 SD below the mean according to the age and education norms instead of at least 1.5 SD per Petersen' criteria); and (c) basic ADLs had to be preserved although more complex ADLs may be slightly impaired (Perneczky, Pohl, Sorg, Hartmann, Komossa et al., 2006). The MCI patients obtained higher scores on the ADAS-Cog scales than the HC ($d = 2.17$), thus showing a greater impairment of cognitive functions (Perneczky, Pohl, Sorg, Hartmann, Komossa et al., 2006). An optimal ADAS-Cog cutoff set at 10 led to satisfying sensitivity and specificity values whereas the discriminating accuracy (AUC = 0.93) was judged excellent (Perneczky, Pohl, Sorg, Hartmann, Komossa et al., 2006).

Table 3. Results of the Studies Assessing the Criterion Validity of the ADAS-Cog for the Detection of MCI

Authors (year)	SAMPLES	Research Design (mean follow-up delay)	RESULTS FROM ROC analyses: Cutoff Sensitivity / Specificity	PPV / NPV (%)	AUC (95% CI)	LR^+ / LR -	OTHER RESULTS	EFFECT SIZE (d) (Total score) 1	2
Class A studies									
Class B studies									
Pyo et al. (2006)	843 HC 135 MCI (CDR= 0.5) 30 AD (CDR= 0.5) 125 AD (CDR= 1)	Cross-sectional controlled	For Tot score: Cutoff = 6: 73% / 89% For Delayed recall: cutoff = 5: 64% / 86%	N/R	N/R	7.09 / 0.24	- MCI > HC on ADAS-Cog Tot and on all subtests	1.74	
Perneczky et al. (2006)	30 HC 45 MCI (CDR= 0.5)	Cross-sectional controlled	Tot optimal cutoff = 10: 78% / 100%	N/R	0.93	6.60 / 0.30	- MCI > HC on ADAS-Cog Tot - ADAS-Cog Tot is a significant predictor of group membership	2.17	

Table 3. (Continued)

Authors (year)	SAMPLES	Research Design (mean follow-up delay)	RESULTS FROM ROC analyses				OTHER RESULTS	EFFECT SIZE (d) (Total score)	
			Cutoff	PPV / NPV	AUC	LR $^{+}$/		1	2
Class C studies									
Grundman et al. (2004)	107 HC 769 MCI 122 AD (CDR= 0.5) 183 AD (CDR= 1.0)	Cross-sectional controlled	N/R	N/R	N/R	N/R	- MCI > HC on ADAS-Cog* Tot, Word list immediate recall, Word list recognition, Without word list items, Word list delayed recall	2.28	
Lam et al. (2005)	78 HC (CDR= 0) 76 QD (CDR= 0.5)	Cross-sectional controlled	N/R	N/R	N/R	N/R	- QD > HC on ADAS-Cog* Tot - ADAS-Cog Tot is a significant predictor of CDR score	1.43	

Note. Class A: Longitudinal (retrospective or prospective) studies that specifically aimed to assess the sensitivity and specificity values of the ADAS-Cog to detect MCI; Class B: Cross-sectional controlled studies that specifically aimed to assess the sensitivity and specificity of the ADAS-Cog to detect the MCI; Class C: Cross-sectional controlled studies comparing the performances of the MCI, other diagnostic groups and/or healthy controls on the ADAS-Cog or prospective longitudinal studies comparing the baseline performances on the ADAS-Cog of MCI who converted with those who did not convert to dementia over time.

PPV = Positive predictive value; NPV = Negative predictive value; AUC = Area under ROC curve; BL = baseline; LR^{+} / LR^{-} = Positive / Negative Likelihood ratios; N/R = Not reported; MCI = Mild Cognitive Impairment; HC = Healthy Controls; AD = Alzheimer's Disease; QD = Questionable Dementia

Convert = MCI converters to dementia; nonConvert = MCI non-converters to dementia

CDR = Clinical Dementia Rating scale score; ADAS-Cog Tot = ADAS-Cog total error score;

* ADAS-Cog Total score is part of the selection procedure for MCI or dementia or is available for diagnosis at baseline (circularity bias)

Effect size[1] = HC vs prevalent MCI ; Effect size[2] = Convert vs Non convert

Finally, a stepwise logistic regression revealed that the ADAS-Cog and the ADSC-MCI-ADL were strong predictors of group membership (Perneczky, Pohl, Sorg, Hartmann, Komossa et al., 2006). The principal limitations of this study are the small sample size and the limited generalization of the findings due to the use of specific criteria for the MCI diagnosis.

Class C Studies

The validity of the ADAS-Cog Total (d = 2.28) and of the memory subtests scores to discriminate MCI-amnesic type patients from the HC was also demonstrated by Grundman et al. (2004) in their Class C study. Like Pyo et al. (2006)'s study, the majority of errors were made by MCI patients on the *Word recall* and *Recognition* items (Grundman et al., 2004). The healthy controls were slightly younger than MCI patients and were less likely to carry the apolipoprotein $E_{\varepsilon 4}$ allele (Grundman et al., 2004). These differences, along with the variables sex, education and race, were controlled for using covariance analyses. The MCI patients also had a statistically significant higher mean score on the Hamilton Depression scale than controls, but it was far from being clinically significant (Grundman et al., 2004). Interestingly, a subset of patients with MCI (25%) had magnetic resonance imaging (MRI) measurements performed at baseline. The results showed that hippocampal volumes were approximately 1 SD below the normal mean, and 0.9 SD larger than those of patients with AD (Grundman et al., 2004). These imaging findings added to the diagnostic validity value of their MCI patients as being in a transitional state between healthy aging and very mild AD. Another strength of this study was the large sample size which allowed sufficient statistical power.

Finally, Lam et al. (2005) compared the neurocognitive profile of 76 Chinese individuals meeting the criteria of questionable dementia (QD) against the profile of 78 HC. Although both QD and HC groups scored above the local cutoff level for dementia, QD patients had lower total ADAS-Cog scores than the HC (Lam et al., 2005). Apart from mentioning the poorer results of the QD compared with the HC participants on the *word list-delayed recall* task, the authors did not provide further details regarding the performance of the participants on the other subtests of the ADAS-Cog. Comparisons of demographical characteristics revealed that the QD patients were significantly older (77.1 ± 6.9 years old) and less educated (2.4 ± 3.8 years of schooling) than the HC (71.9 ± 7.2 years old and 5.0 ± 4.4 years of schooling) (Lam et al., 2005). The authors did not control for these confounding variables which could explained the forehead results. Nevertheless, age and education level were considered in a backward stepwise logistic regression analysis, along with other significant variables affecting CDR grouping. Only the ADAS-Cog total score, *Reverse Visual Span* and *Category Verbal Fluency* Tests were retained as significant predictors of the CDR grouping.

Discussion of the ADAS-Cog Results

The evidence regarding the criterion validity of the ADAS-Cog for the detection of MCI comes from only four cross-sectional studies, using different diagnostic criteria for MCI (see the QD criteria and the Petersen's MCI criteria). The cohort effect could not be ruled out for explaining the results. Moreover, the absence of longitudinal data prevents the confirmation of an eventual conversion from MCI to dementia. Only the study of Grundman et al. (2006)

provided some convergent MRI data supporting their MCI grouping as a prodromal phase of dementia. Pyo et al. (2006) demonstrated that unlike healthy elderly individuals and AD patients, the educational level did account for the ADAS-Cog total score in the MCI population. This finding needs to be replicated. In addition, there was clearly a ceiling effect on all the non-memory subtests of the ADAS-Cog (Grundman et al., 2004; Pyo et al., 2006). Taken into account that only a proportion of patients will present with an initial memory impairment (Peterson and Morris, 2003), it is mandatory to revise the non-memory subtests to improve their sensitivity to measure cognitive changes in patients with MCI and early AD (Pyo et al., 2006). Nevertheless, the ADAS-Cog seems to be a promising tool, at least in clinical setting. Indeed, the LR^+ values are substantially higher for the ADAS-Cog than for the MMSE, suggesting that the ADAS-Cog seems to be a better instrument in screening people with MCI. However, its sensitivity still remains to be addressed in a more general setting.

Mattis Dementia Rating Scale (MDRS)

Brief Description of the Instrument

The Mattis Dementia Rating Scale (MDRS) was initially developed for the assessment and follow-up of cognitively impaired individuals, principally suffering from a cortical neurodegenerative disease (Coblentz et al., 1973; Mattis, 1976). The MDRS was designed to provide an overall score of cognitive deficits based upon performances on a variety of cognitive tasks regrouped in five subtests: *Attention*, *Initiation/Perseveration*, *Construction*, *Conceptualization* and *Memory*. The total maximum score is 144, and the scoring system is positive. The Table 4 presents all the items included in each subscale and their respective maximum score.

Table 4. Description of the five subscales of the Mattis Dementia Rating Scale

MDRS Subscales (maximum score)	Items (number of points)
Attention (37)	Digit span (8); Two-step commands (2); One-step commands (4); Imitation of commands (4); Counting A's (6); Counting randomly arranged A's (5); Read a word list (4) and Match figures (4).
Initiation / Perseveration (37)	Fluency for supermarket items (20); Fluency for clothing items (8); Verbal repetition (e.g. bee, key, gee) (2); Double alternating movements (3) and Graphomotor (copy alternating figures) (4).
Construction (6)	Copy geometric designs (5) and Writing your name (1).
Conceptualization (39)	Similarities (8); Priming inductive reasoning (3); Detection of different items (3); Multiple choice similarities (8); Identities and oddities (16) and Create a sentence (1).
Memory (25)	Recall a sentence (4); Recall a self-generated sentence (3); Orientation (e.g. place, date) (9); Verbal recognition (5) and Figure recognition (4).

The items of the MDRS are presented in a hierarchical manner. This way, a correct answer to the first items of a subtest allows the examiner to give credits for the subsequent items. For this reason, the administration lasts from 10 to 15 minutes in elderly people without cognitive deficits, and from 30 to 45 minutes in severely impaired individuals.

Previous studies demonstrated the temporal stability of the MDRS in a normal population (Smith et al., 1994) as well as its sensitivity to cognitive deterioration, in patients with dementia (Smith et al., 1994) and A-MCI (Chetelat et al., 2005). These qualities are particularly useful in the early detection of a neurodegenerative disease and its follow-up (Franzen, 2000). On the other hand, some data revealed that the MDRS total score was significantly associated with age and education level (Freidl et al., 2002; Schmidt et al., 1994; Vangel and Lichtenberg, 1995). Race and gender are not associated nor could predict the MDRS total score in several studies (Marcopulos, McLain, and Giuliano, 1997; Monsch et al., 1995; Woodard, Auchus, Godsall, and Green, 1998). However, other studies indicated that there could be a cultural bias or educational differences in severely impaired AD Hispanic patients (Hohl, Grundman, Salmon, Thomas, and Thal, 1999), and in elderly Chinese individuals (Chan, Choi, and Salmon, 2001).

Regarding the criterion validity, it is well established than the MDRS can distinguish between mild to moderate AD and healthy elderly individuals (Green, Woodard, and Green, 1995; Monsch et al., 1995; Vitaliano et al., 1984). Several studies also revealed cognitive and qualitative differences between AD and other neurodegenerative syndromes involving cortical and / or subcortical alterations such as fronto-temporal dementia (Rascovsky et al., 2002), Huntington's disease (Paulsen et al., 1995; Rosser and Hodges, 1994; Salmon, Kwo-on-Yuen, Heindel, Butters, and Thal, 1989), progressive supranuclear palsy (Aarsland et al., 2003; Rosser and Hodges, 1994), Parkinson's disease with and without dementia (Aarsland et al., 2003; Paolo, Troster, Glatt, Hubble, and Koller, 1995), and dementia with Lewy bodies. Nevertheless, the capacity of the MDRS to differentially diagnose MCI from HC and AD is still unknown.

Review of the Studies Assessing the Criterion Validity of the MDRS for the Detection of MCI

Only three studies were found to provide some information regarding the criterion validity of the MDRS to detect MCI (see Table 5). A cross-sectional controlled study (Boeve et al., 2003), and a prospective longitudinal study (Griffith et al., 2006) were categorized in Class C, whereas our cross-sectional controlled study was classified in Class B (Matteau and colleagues).

Class B Study

The goal of our cross-sectional controlled study was to investigate the criterion validity of the MDRS. We retrospectively analyzed the data included in a non nominative computerized database created at the *Laboratoire de Recherche en Neuropsychologie Gériatrique* at Laval University, Quebec City, Canada. All subjects were 50 years old and greater, and they had been recruited both in community and specialized memory disorder clinics in the Canadian provinces of Quebec, Ontario and New Brunswick to participate in studies on normal and pathological aging.

Each of these studies had previously been approved by the Ethics Committees where the research took place. In all cases, the participants were administered an exhaustive neuropsychological evaluation including the MDRS. Twenty-one individuals met the A-MCI criteria (Petersen et al., 2004), 23 met the NINDS-ADRDA (McKhann et al., 1984) and DSM-IV (APA, 1994) criteria for probable AD, and 28 participants were healthy elderly controls. In order to be included in the A-MCI group, the patients had to present a significant and predominant episodic memory deficit (approximately 1.5 SD or more below the mean per the normative sample) on the list learning (trials 1 to 5) or delayed free recall parameters of the California Verbal Learning Test (CVLT) (Delis, Kramer, Kaplan, and Ober, 1987), and to perform relatively within normal limits on the tasks of other cognitive domains (≥ -1.0 SD).

All statistical analyses were conducted using the SPSS program for Windows version 11.0. Alpha level was set at .05 for first level analyses. In order to reduce the Type I error, post hoc group comparisons were corrected using the Bonferroni procedure. Table 6 presents the demographical characteristics of each group.

The first level ANOVA analyses revealed that the groups were not equivalent on age (F (2, 69) = 12.81, $p < .0001$) and education level (F (2, 69) = 8.53, $p < .0001$). As indicated by post hoc multiple comparisons, this multivariate effect was principally due to the AD patients who were significantly older ($p \leq .001$) and less educated ($p \leq .006$) than the other groups. However, the proportion of women was similar (χ^2 (2, N = 72) = 2.23, p = .33) in the three groups of participants. The performances of each group on the five MDRS subtests, and the effect size for all possible contrasts are reported in Table 7.

All groups were different on the MDRS age- and education-corrected scaled total score (F (2, 69)= 176.39, $p < .0001$). A MANCOVA, applied to age-corrected scaled scores with the educational level as covariable, showed that at least two groups were also distinct on all subtests (F (6, 63)= 63.35, $p < .0001$). Post hoc pairwise comparisons confirmed that AD patients performed significantly worse than the other groups on the MDRS Total and all the subtests scores (all $p < .0001$). The patients with MCI scored significantly lower than the HC on the MDRS total score and on the *Initiation/Perseveration* (p = .038) and *Memory* subscales (p = .001). Finally, the A-MCI group performed consistently better than the AD group (p = .000), except on the *Attention* subscale (p = .012).

In order to determine which variables could better differentiate the three groups, a discriminant function analysis (DFA), stepwise forward method (F to enter = .05, F to remove = .10) was computed. Age, education and age-corrected scaled scores of the five MDRS subscales were entered as potential contributory variables. The MDRS total score was not included to avoid redundancy (matrix ill-conditioning problem). The results showed that only one discriminant function provided an optimal discrimination between the three groups. The best discriminators were the performances on *Memory* (step 1), *Initiation/Perseveration* (step 2) and *Construction* (step 3) subscales. Canonical correlation for the equation including these three variables was .94. Then, a classification analysis based upon *Memory*, Initiation/Perseveration and Construction subtests demonstrated an overall classification accuracy of 84.7%, with 85.7% of the HC group, 66.7% of the A-MCI group and 100% of the AD group being correctly classified.

Table 5. Results of the Studies Assessing the Criterion Validity of the MDRS for the Detection of MCI

Authors (year)	SAMPLES	Research Device (mean follow-up delay)	RESULTS FROM ROC analyses: Cutoff Sensitivity / Specificity	PPV / NPV (%)	AUC (95% CI)	LR $^{+}$ / LR -	OTHER RESULTS	EFFECT SIZE (*d*) (Total score) 1	2
Class A studies									
Class B studies									
Matteau *et al.* (original data)	28 HC 21 A-MCI 23 AD	Cross-sectional	Optimal cutoff = 138: 71.4% / 67.9%	N/R	0.78 (.64 - .92)	2.22 / 0.42	- A-MCI < HC on MDRS* Tot and on Mem and I/P subscales	1.1[a]	
Class C studies									
Griffith *et al.* (2006)	49 HC 49 A-MCI (CDR= 0.5)	Prospective Longitudinal (1.1 year)	N/R	N/R	N/R	N/R	- MCI < HC on BL MDRS* Tot and on Mem and I/P subtests - Follow-up: 13 Convert vs 36 nonConvert - Convert = nonConvert on MDRS Tot and on all subscales - MDRS I/P subtest is a significant predictor of conversion to AD	0.90	0.87

Table 5. (Continued)

Authors (year)	SAMPLES	Research Device (mean follow-up delay)	RESULTS FROM ROC analyses				OTHER RESULTS	EFFECT SIZE (*d*) (Total score)	
			Cutoff	PPV / NPV	AUC	LR $^{+}$/		1	2
Class C studies									
Boeve *et al.* (2003)	56 HC 13 A-MCI 42 degenerative dementia	Cross-sectional	N/R	N/R	N/R	N/R	- A-MCI = HC on MDRS Tot - A-MCI < HC on Mem subscale	1.20	

Note. Class A: Longitudinal (retrospective or prospective) studies that specifically aimed to assess the sensitivity and specificity values of the MDRS to detect MCI; Class B: Cross-sectional controlled studies that specifically aimed to assess the sensitivity and specificity of the MDRS to detect MCI; Class C: Cross-sectional controlled studies comparing the performances of the MCI, other diagnostic groups and/or healthy controls on the MDRS or prospective longitudinal studies comparing the baseline performances on the MDRS of MCI who converted and those who did not convert to dementia over time.

PPV = Positive predictive value; NPV = Negative predictive value; AUC = Area under ROC curve; BL = baseline; LR^{+} / LR^{-} = Positive / Negative Likelihood ratios; N/R = Not reported; A-MCI = Amnesic Mild Cognitive Impairment; HC = Healthy Controls; AD = Alzheimer's Disease

Convert = MCI converters to dementia; nonConvert = MCI non-converters to dementia

CDR = Clinical Dementia Rating scale score; MDRS Tot = Mattis Dementia Rating Scale total score; I/P = Initiation/Perseveration; Mem = Memory

* MDRS Total score is part of the selection procedure for MCI or dementia or is available for diagnosis at baseline (circularity bias)

Effect size[1] = HC vs prevalent MCI Effect size[2] = Convert vs nonConvert

[a] Effect size was calculated using age- and education-corrected scaled scores

Table 6. Means (M) and Standard Deviations (SD) of the Demographic Data

	Diagnostic groups					
	Healthy Controls $n = 28$		A-MCI $n = 21$		AD $n = 23$	
Variable	M	(SD)	M	(SD)	M	(SD)
Age[a]	69.9	(9.3)	66.0	(8.8)	79.0	(8.3)
Education[b] (years completed)	14.3	(3.2)	12.2	(4.2)	10.5	(2.9)
Sex (% women)	60.7%		52.3%		73.9%	

[a] AD > A-MCI and Healthy Controls ($p < .001$); [b] AD < A-MCI and Healthy controls ($p < .006$).

Table 7. Performances and effect size observed between the groups on MDRS subscales and Total scores

	DIAGNOSTIC GROUPS					
	HC $n = 28$	A-MCI $n = 21$	AD $n = 23$	Effect size (d)[a]		
MDRS	M (SD)	M (SD)	M (SD)	1-2	1-3	2-3
Attention	12.9 (0.9)	11.9 (1.2)	10.3 (2.3)	0.9	1.6	1.5
Initiation/Perseveration	10.2 (1.6)	8.6 (2.8)	3.3 (1.7)	0.7	4.1	3.0
Construction	9.1 (1.4)	9.6 (1.1)	6.1 (2.9)	-0.4	1.4	1.5
Abstraction	10.9 (1.7)	9.9 (1.9)	5.3 (2.6)	0.5	2.6	2.5
Memory	12.2 (1.7)	10.1 (2.8)	2.6 (1.5)	0.9	6.2	4.5
Total (SS)	11.9 (1.8)	9.3 (2.7)	2.0 (1.1)	1.2	6.8	3.8
Total (raw score)	140.1 (2.6)	136.0 (4.6)	100.9 (13.6)	1.3	4.8	3.9

Note. Values are age-corrected scaled score (SS) for all subscales and age- and education-corrected scaled scores (SS) for the MDRS Total.

[a] 1 = HC; 2 = A-MCI; 3 = AD.

Because it has been argued that multilinearity between neuropsychological measures could lead to instability of the analyses performed (Tian et al., 2003), we conducted another DFA, this time using the Enter method, in order to explore the stability of our discriminant model. The results showed that the same three variables significantly contributed to the differentiation between the three groups.

A DFA was then conducted for the outcome classification HC versus MCI using the variables which were found significantly different between these two groups. The discriminant model based upon *Initiation/Perseveration* and *Memory* subtests age-corrected scaled scores showed 67% sensitivity and 86% specificity ($LR^+ = 4.8$, $LR^- = .38$). Finally, a ROC analysis was used to assess the accuracy of the MDRS as a screen test to detect MCI. Keeping the sensitivity / specificity optimal, the best cutoff was established at 138 out of 144. Corresponding sensitivity, specificity and LR values are shown in Table 5.

The total score and all subscales of the MDRS properly distinguished AD from HC, and AD from A-MCI (except for the *Attention* subtest). However, only the *Initiation/Perseveration* and the *Memory* subscales differentiated A-MCI patients from HC. These subtests, combined with the *Construction* subtest, were also the best discriminators of group membership with an overall classification of 84.7%. The current results were congruent with prior research showing that cognitive tests tapping into episodic memory and executive functions are amongst the first to show deterioration long before dementia symptoms become clinically apparent (Saxton et al., 2004). Structural and functional neuroimaging studies in preclinical AD could offer a neuranatomical and neurophysiological rationale for the present neuropsychological results. Indeed, longitudinal studies have demonstrated that decreased enthorinal cortex volume and atrophy can predict which patients with MCI will develop AD (deToledo-Morrell et al., 2004; Dickerson et al., 2001). The enthorinal cortex is located in the anterior parahippocampal gyrus and is well recognized to be involved in episodic memory (Gomez-Isla et al., 1996). SPECT studies also have shown that reduced cerebral blood flow in cingulate and left frontal regions are predictive of progression to AD (Cabranes et al., 2004; Nestor, Scheltens, and Hodges, 2004). These results may explain, in part, the alteration of both memory and executive functioning in early AD (Albert, Moss, Tanzi, and Jones, 2001; Arikuni, Sako, and Murata, 1994).

Pertaining to methodology, this study is, with Tabert et al. (2006)'s, the first to use results corrected for age and education level before performing any statistical analyses. Despite its strengths and interesting findings, this study had some limitations. Because the clinicians who made the diagnosis of MCI were not blind to the results of the MDRS, there was a risk of circularity bias. However, the MDRS results were not used as inclusion / exclusion criteria for the diagnostic groups; the performances on the CVLT, overall cognitive assessment, input of the informant, and clinical judgment were instead specifically considered for this purpose. Other limitations included the utilization of a retrospective and cross-sectional experimental design as well as the absence of postmortem histopathological confirmation of AD. In such cases, the cognitive profile of the A-MCI patients observed on the MDRS could not yet be considered specifically as a prodrome of AD.

Class C Studies

In order to examine the clinical, demographic and neuropsychological predictors of conversion to probable AD dementia, 49 patients newly diagnosed with MCI and 49 HC were followed for a two-year period (Griffith et al., 2006). The MCI diagnosis was based on Petersen et al. (2001)'s criteria for the amnesic type. The MDRS was part of an extensive neuropsychological battery. Applying the Bonferroni procedure (α = .002) for multiple comparisons, the statistical analysis showed that the MCI group had lower scores at baseline than HC on the MDRS total score and *Memory* subscale. At one-year follow-up, 11 of the 49 A-MCI patients developed AD. Amongst the 17 participants with a two-year follow-up, two converted to AD for an average annual conversion rate of 17.11%. Analyses of variance performed between converters and non-converters to dementia on their baseline characteristics and neuropsychological scores showed that the only significant difference was for the use of cholinesterase inhibitors. These nootropics were more frequently prescribed to converters than non-converters. Using a less conservative method (α = .01), a trend towards significance was observed for group differences on MDRS-*Memory* and *Initiation/Perseveration* subtests and the Wechsler Memory Scale III-Visual Reproduction II and Percent Retention (Griffith et al., 2006). These measures were included in a stepwise discriminant function analysis in order to identify the best predictor of group status at follow-up. A model based on Visual Reproduction Percent Retention and MDRS *Initiation/Perseveration* scores correctly classified 85.7% of the MCI sample as either converters or non-converters (Griffith et al., 2006). The short follow-up period was a problem in this study since it is possible that the non-converter group included patients who later developed dementia. The small sample size at the entry of the study may have induced a lack of statistical power for the analyses performed on the baseline results of converters versus non-converters at follow-up. In addition, as usual in cross-sectional and short longitudinal studies, the absence of a neuropathological confirmation of the AD diagnosis constituted another difficulty.

Boeve et al. (2003) performed comprehensive neurological, functional, and neuropsychological assessments, including the MDRS, in an attempt to verify if the syndrome of A-MCI occurs in the oldest old, i.e. in individuals aged 90 years and greater. Thirteen persons presented with A-MCI, 42 with degenerative dementia, and 56 were healthy controls. The A-MCI patients scored, in average, eight points under the HC, but this difference was not statistically significant. Nevertheless, the *Memory* subscale was useful to differentiate between the groups ($d = 1.40$). A weaker performance of the very old controls (compared to old controls) might have restricted the extent of further decline in MCI patients, and might thus explain the non significant results (Backman et al., 2004). In addition, the small number of participants with A-MCI may perhaps have limited the possibility of finding a significant difference on the MDRS-total score because of a lack of statistical power.

Discussion of the MDRS Results

The paucity of data on the criterion validity of the MDRS precludes a definite conclusion regarding the sensitivity value of this cognitive measure to the presence of MCI. The two Class C studies were not designed to investigate this important question, and the Class B study was not longitudinal. Nevertheless, their preliminary results provided some interesting findings, underscoring the importance of the *Memory* and, to a lesser extent, the *Initiation/Perseveration* subtests, to differentiate MCI from healthy elderly, even in the oldest old. The same subtests properly differentiated the MCI patients who converted to dementia from those who remained stable (Griffith et al., 2006). In addition, our results (Class B study) showed that the MDRS age- and education-corrected total score was useful to detect MCI. However, our data combined with those of Griffith et al. (2006) strongly suggested that *Attention* and *Construction* subtests should be modified in order to increase their level of difficulty because of a ceiling effect.

General Discussion

The main objective of this chapter was to critically review some of the most widely used cognitive screening tests with a particular emphasis on their efficacy to detect MCI individuals. As expected, the MMSE was the most studied. We indeed reported the findings from 28 studies, 18 of them focusing on the MMSE, three on the CAMCOG, four on the ADAS-Cog, and three on the MDRS.

The findings regarding the criterion validity of the MMSE for preclinical AD were quite inconsistent. The effect size varied from 0.32 (small to moderate) to 5.94 (large) between HC and MCI scores, and from 0.13 (small) to 2.00 (large) between MCI non-converters and MCI converters to dementia. Despite a moderate-to-large effect size in some studies, a careful observation of raw scores revealed important overlaps between the groups. An examination of the likelihood ratios strongly suggested that the clinical utility of the MMSE was lower in community-dwelling people than in patients from clinical settings. Because individuals noticing memory difficulties are in general more likely to attend specialized clinics (Feldman and Jacova, 2005), they are also more likely to present at a more advanced stage of cognitive decline (Lehrner et al., 2005). However, the contribution of the MMSE in the diagnostic process of MCI still appeared to be limited in the present review.

Despite some limitations (see the above section), the MDRS certainly has some advantages compared to the other screening tests reviewed. These advantages might explain the consistent results of the MDRS in the three studies reviewed in this chapter, and reporting some positive results on the sensitivity of the *Memory* and *Initiation/Perseveration* subscales to distinguish A-MCI from HC. The MDRS has been reported in previous research to be more detailed and sensitive than the MMSE to early AD-associated cognitive changes, particularly with repeated measurements (Salmon, Thal, Butters, and Heindel, 1990). Compared to the MMSE, it offers the advantage of measuring several cognitive functions with multiple items and hence, provides estimates of the relative contribution of each cognitive function to global score changes (Chetelat et al., 2005). Contrary to the CAMCOG and ADAS-Cog, the MDRS assesses executive functions such as verbal and motor initiation through the *Initiation/Perseveration* subscale. Approximately 75% of this subtest reflects verbal fluency abilities which imply both executive functioning (initiation and retrieval strategies) and semantic memory (see Table 4). Along with an episodic memory deficit, semantic memory is one of the first cognitive spheres affected in preclinical AD (Feldman and Jacova, 2005).

On the other hand, the different episodic memory processes (encoding, retrieval, consolidation) are certainly best evaluated using the ADAS-Cog provided that a delayed recall paradigm is added. However, this is at the cost of a longer administration time which is certainly not an asset in a screening context.

Finally, one should acknowledge the practice effects arising from multiple expositions to the test considering that most MCI patients will undergo several follow-up cognitive assessments until a diagnosis of dementia will be made. The MDRS is the only screening measure for which an alternate form is available, thus allowing serial administrations within a relatively brief period of time. This might certainly contribute obtaining a better classification of cognitive decline (Schmidt, Mattis, Adams, and Nestor, 2005b).

In order to achieve the detection of MCI and prediction of future progression to AD, discriminant or regression models were proposed by several groups of authors (Griffith et al., 2006; Isella et al., 2006; Jelle Visser, Verhey, Jolles, and Jonker, 2002; Li et al., 2006; Perneczky, Pohl, Sorg, Hartmann, Komossa et al., 2006; Tian et al., 2003). Some of these models resulted in satisfying sensitivity and overall classification of MCI, HC and AD. However, the real test for a given model comes when it is applied on different data, i.e. on a different sample from which the model was computed. Thus, these suggested models will need to be further validated in new cases.

Methodological Considerations

There are many possible reasons to explain inconsistency in the magnitude of the findings between the studies, especially in regards to the MMSE studies. Characteristics of the population screened are amongst the first to consider. Because performances on all the tests reviewed are influenced by age and education (Lezak, 1995; Lezak et al., 2004), differences between diagnostic groups on these two variables cannot be ignored. To avoid such differences, the first solution is to match controls to patients on relevant variables at entry of the study. If group matching isn't possible and comparisons between groups reveal significant differences on age and / or education, it is recommended to statistically control *a posteriori* for these differences in order to minimize confounding noise (Kazdin, 2003). Despite the well-established influence of age and education on neuropsychological performances, only a few authors considered it as an alternative explanation for the differences observed between MCI and HC on the cognitive screening measure. On the other hand, it has been suggested that effect sizes between cognitive scores of cases and controls tend to be larger for earlier onset (< 75 years) than for later onset (> 75 years) of MCI (Backman et al., 2004). After verification of our findings on the screening tests reviewed, we did not observe increased effect sizes as a function of earlier onset. Moreover, the results did not seem to vary according to the mean educational level or the population screened (community-dwelling versus clinical). However, all these characteristics interact with each other and more research is required to determine the influence of these respective interacting factors on the findings.

One should also acknowledge that the different diagnostic criteria and / or psychometric definitions of MCI used by various teams of researchers might explain some discrepancy between the results in the studies reviewed. Apart from Petersen's (2000; 2004) conceptualization of MCI, some authors, using the CAMCOG and the ADAS-Cog (see Tables 2 and 3) employed a different definition such as minimal dementia or questionable dementia (QD). Despite the fact that the three concepts share similar characteristics, they should not be considered as equivalent. For example, the term minimal dementia comes from the CAMDEX nomenclature and its diagnosis is made according to overall clinical impression when the patients do not reach the strict criteria of dementia (per the DSM-IV for example), but present with a limited and variable impairment in cognitive impairment (in memory and other cognitive domains), as well as in daily living (Roth et al., 1986). Although the most widespread, the definition elaborated par Petersen (2001; 2004) has been criticized for a lack of operationalized criteria (Luis et al., 2003). This is particularly obvious in regards to the abnormal memory criteria. Petersen (2001) mentioned that the score on the memory task should be «generally» 1.5 SD or more below the mean per age-appropriate norms. However, he did not yet specify which memory test is the most appropriate nor did he clarify on which paradigm (encoding, delayed recall, recognition) the patient is expected to be impaired. Consequently, it becomes the researcher's responsibility to decide how to apply the criteria. Therefore, a variety of memory tests are used and the severity of the deficit isn't homogeneous from one study to the other. In addition, it is not unusual for researchers to use a Clinical Dementia Rating (CDR) (Hughes et al., 1982) score of 0.5 as an inclusion criteria for their participants with A-MCI. This is self-contradictory because a CDR of 0.5 embraces elderly people with a more heterogeneous cognitive state than A-MCI. Indeed, apart from minor impairment in orientation and memory, subjects with a CDR 0.5 may also have a slight impairment or deterioration in judgement and community skills (Collie and Maruff, 2002; Lam et al., 2005).

Independent of the definition (MCI, minimal dementia or QD) adopted by the authors, the use of a score of CDR 0.5 as an inclusion criteria is particularly frequent when studying people at risk of evolving towards dementia. However, it has already been demonstrated that AD-specific pathologic markers could be found in most CDR 0.5 cases (Morris et al., 2001), and that about a third of patients with CDR 0.5 are diagnosable as very mild AD patients (Petersen and Morris, 2003). Consequently, if one is interested in investigating the prodromal phase of dementia, including patients with CDR 0.5 is not recommended otherwise the MCI sample may include people with very early dementia, and thus bias the findings.

Many studies revealed the ability of all the cognitive measures under review to detect, at some point, the presence of MCI. This is first noticeable on the total score which could reflect the actual global cognitive functioning of the patient. The notion of multiple cognitive system breakdown in preclinical AD gives an interpretation framework to this finding (Backman et al., 2004; Backman, Jones, Berger, Laukka, and Small, 2005). When subscales scores or items were analysed, those covering episodic memory emerged as the most sensitive to MCI (see the results of the CAMCOG, ADAS-Cog and MDRS). The degree of confidence for this finding is, somehow, limited. Indeed, since MCI is in itself defined by cognitive dysfunction and, for the most part by memory impairment, it is practically impossible to rule out circularity bias as a potential explanation for this result. This may be true even when there is no cross-contamination between neuropsychological results and clinical diagnosis (Feldman and Jacova, 2005). Circularity bias is a major problem in Class C studies, but also in Class B studies, when MCI is predefined using neuropsychological test results, and then similar outcome measures are used. In addition, the other cognitive functions are somehow, not well measured in screening tests, especially in the ADAS-Cog, CAMCOG and MMSE, thus enhancing the probability of finding a significant effect on memory subtasks. Nevertheless, Petersen and O'Brien (2006) emphasized that MCI should not be only a neuropsychological diagnosis, and that its determination lies on the clinician's judgment in the same way as one would make the diagnosis of dementia or AD.

The disparity in conversion rates from MCI to dementia has pointed out the unstable nature of MCI (Larrieu et al., 2002). The reversion rates to normality vary from 6% (Isella et al., 2006; Tian et al., 2003) to as much as 40% (Larrieu et al., 2002). Diagnosis of MCI based solely on the performance on a single measure (cutoff score) can lead to inherent instability in the outcome by neglecting the potential etiologies of the cognitive impairment (Petersen and O'Brien, 2006). Because there are many explanations for changes in cognitive status (e.g., neurodegenerative disease, infection, metabolic changes, depression, medication side effects), a proper documentation of symptom progression is imperative for an accurate diagnosis (Schmidt, Mattis, Adams, and Nestor, 2005a). Given the absence of an actual gold standard for MCI, the predictive validity of MCI for clinical dementia should be the basis for its definition (Ganguli, Dodge et al., 2004; Petersen and O'Brien, 2006). However, the unique way to ensure that MCI is truly preclinical AD (or another dementia), is to follow patients until a definite diagnosis can be made (Xu et al., 2002).

When the time comes to compare results between the studies, we are confronted to the various baseline-to-follow-up periods that may also have contributed to the variable outcomes. The mean follow-up duration of studies under review was less than three years after the baseline assessment. At this point in time, it is still unclear when exactly a precipitous cognitive decline generally occurs in preclinical AD (Backman et al., 2004). Given that the neurocellular changes associated with AD can be detected many years before clinical onset (Grady et al., 1988), this cast doubt on the extent to which MCI participants were really «not demented» at baseline. Moreover, regarding the low base rate of dementia in the general population, a large sample size is needed at baseline to optimize statistical power requirements (Kazdin, 2003). This condition is rarely met.

One of the limitations of the longitudinal studies is that a certain number of subjects recruited at baseline had no follow-up assessment, which is common in community-based studies on elderly subjects (Luis et al., 2003). The loss of subjects reduces the sample size, thus limiting the statistical power and the magnitude of the effect size observed (Kazdin, 2003). This could lead to erroneous conclusions about the absence of effect when it is otherwise present (Kazdin, 2003). Most importantly, the attrition problem lies in its selectivity, which makes the groups non equivalent on characteristics potentially relevant to the results (Cotter, Burke, Loeber, and Navratil, 2002). The issue of attrition is often neglected.. In the studies reviewed, a few investigators addressed the question by comparing, on several baseline variables, drop-out and / or lost participants with those who stayed. According to Streiner (2002), even this procedure is insufficient because the absence of difference could still come from the lack of statistical power. Other variables not measured or interactions between variables could also be responsible for the loss of subjects. Thus, even if no differences between the two groups are found on baseline characteristics, it still remains possible that a selective attrition occurred (Streiner, 2002). The choice of appropriate statistical tests to control *a posteriori* for the attrition problem is also important. Methods like Cox regression (survival analysis) (Tian et al., 2003) or random effect models (Petkova and Teresi, 2002) allow to model time to event data that can account for censored cases. Nevertheless, researchers should develop retention strategies at the time of the project elaboration.

Clinical Considerations

The interpretation of a screening measure should rely on an understanding of the meaning of an individual score which, in return, is influenced by the goal of the examination and the reference population of the patient (Meiran et al., 1996; Strauss et al., 2006). The use of cutoff scores to determine if a pathological condition might be present or absent is widespread in clinical settings. However, this dichotomous way of interpretation (affected or not affected) does not take into account that the same score might be obtained both by subjects with and without the disease. In addition, a cutoff taken alone oversimplifies the screening context by not accounting for the prevalence of dementia in a particular setting (Derogatis and Lynn, 2000; Meiran et al., 1996). The use of cutoff scores is therefore not recommended (Derogatis and Lynn, 2000; Meiran et al., 1996). Typical prevalence values for dementia are 2% (community, ages 64-75 years), 10% (medical inpatients), 20% (community, ages 74-85 years), 50% (community older than 85 years and nursing homes) and 75% (memory clinics) (Meiran et al., 1996). Prevalence rates of predementia syndromes are less well established and vary largely as a result of different diagnostic criteria as well as different sampling and assessment procedures (Panza et al., 2005). Nevertheless, prevalence of MCI has been estimated from 3.2% (Ganguli, Dodge et al., 2004) to 19% (Lopez et al., 2003) in population-based studies, and is reported to be higher in clinical-referred samples (Feldman and Jacova, 2005). Prevalence of MCI also increases as a function of older age (Feldman and Jacova,

2005; Graham, Cully, Snow, Massman, and Doody, 2004; Graham et al., 1997; Lopez et al., 2003).

No matter what the base rates are, likelihood ratios may improve clinical certainty that a disease is present or absent. As described earlier, the LR can be computed from the sensitivity / specificity values of a test, and give relevant information about the probability of the disease associated with a particular test result (Jaeschke et al., 2002). Moreover, LR can adapt results from a study to a patient according to Bayes' theorem, which is a mathematical relationship describing how a diagnostic finding changes our knowledge of the probability of abnormality (Sackett, Straus, Richardson, Rosenberg, and Haynes, 2000). Thus, LR can be used as an adjustment factor to convert a pre-test probability (or pre-test odds) into a post-test probability (or post-test odds). The formula for post-test odds is the following:

Post-test odds = Pre-test odds x LR,

where the pre-test odds represents the chances that the person has the disease based only on the knowledge about the existing prevalence data regarding the particular clinical setting in which the screening occurs. Knowing the LR^+ and / or the LR^-, the post-test odds reflects the adjusted probability that a given patient has the disease taking into account the prevalence base rate of the disease (Meiran et al., 1996). In order to propose a convenient way to estimate the post-test probability, Fagan (1975) has developed a likelihood ratio nomogram derived from Bayes' theorem. The Fagan's, or other similar nomograms, are easily available in books on critical appraisal. Many calculators are also forthcoming on the web.

In clinical practice, knowing how a test result predicts the risk of abnormality is particularly important. Sensitivity and specificity values do the reverse: they provide information about how abnormality (or normality) can predict test results. Predictive values (PPV, NPV) do give probabilities of abnormality for particular test results. However, they are influenced by the prevalence of a pathological condition in the study sample and can rarely be generalized beyond the study (except when the study is conducted on a suitable random sample, like in some population screening studies) (Deeks and Altman, 2004; Warner, 2004). Likelihood ratios consist of a more flexible solution as they can be employed to compute the probability of abnormality, while adapting for different prior probabilities according to various contexts (Deeks and Altman, 2004). Consequently, authors should provide sufficient data to calculate sensitivity, specificity, and LR to be applied in clinical practice.

Recommendations for Future Research

The lack of consensus regarding the applicability of the MCI research-based concept in clinical practice, the heterogeneity of cognitive deficits in MCI and its prognosis (evolutive, stable, reversible) have raised some doubts about the clinical significance of MCI in elderly people (Alladi, Arnold, Mitchell, Nestor, and Hodges, 2006). Given the high prevalence of AD, the major interest of researchers was primarily and principally directed at the examination of MCI as a potential risk factor for its development. The amnesic-type MCI was long considered to be the prodromal phase of AD (Petersen, 2004). Nevertheless and unlike previously stated, increasing evidence argues that pure amnesic MCI is rare when using more stringent psychometric tests, and the patients with A-MCI could in fact present with subtle impairments in other cognitive domains (Alladi et al., 2006; Grundman et al., 2004; Hodges et al., 2006). Apart from an episodic memory decline, a meta-analysis has revealed marked preclinical deficits in perceptual speed and executive functioning (Backman et al., 2005). This strongly suggests that the objective assessment of MCI should encompass multiple cognitive domains, and not be concentrated only on memory function, especially when using a screening test. This could help to identify a subgroup of MCI sufferers who are cognitively more at risk to develop clinical dementia (Lam et al., 2005). Thus, a good screening test should cover these cognitive domains relevant to the diagnosis of MCI through multiple items, and with sufficient variability in difficulty to ensure a satisfactory level of sensitivity.

According to the Petersen et al. (2001) definition, MCI is separated from mild dementia by the preserved capacity to perform daily living activities. Certain researchers have expressed some doubts about the validity of this criteria (Perneczky, Pohl, Sorg, Hartmann, Komossa et al., 2006; Tabert et al., 2002). Indeed, there is some evidence that more complex activities involving memory or complex reasoning, such as organizing work and managing finances, may be by particularly impaired in MCI patients compared to HC whereas more basic activities, such as bathing and getting dressed, remain unaffected (Perneczky, Pohl, Sorg, Hartmann, Tosic et al., 2006). Another study revealed that baseline self- and informant-reported functional deficits may help to predict which patients will convert to AD at follow-up evaluation, and which patients will not, even after controlling for age, education, and modified Mini-Mental State Examination score (Tabert et al., 2002). Consequently, complex ADLs could be more routinely assessed given their probable utility for the diagnosis of MCI.

Studies on the capacity of screening tests to detect MCI and to predict conversion to AD have given mixed results. The utilization of convergent screening methods such as informant reports (Tierney, Herrmann, Geslani, and Szalai, 2003) or brief functional assessments (Perneczky, Pohl, Sorg, Hartmann, Komossa et al., 2006), and other cognitive (Tierney et al., 2003) or clinical (e.g. ApoEε4 genotype) (Lee, 2006) measures are proposed to improve the prediction of future dementia (predictive validity). There is evidence that the efficacy of detecting persons at risk to develop AD is substantially increased when neuropsycholoical tasks evaluating different cognitive functions are combined into the same prediction model (Bozoki et al., 2001). For example, when considering the additive predictive value of clear cognitive impairments beyond memory loss (e.g. verbal ability) at baseline in patients with MCI, it has been shown that the risk of dementia over a three-year period is significantly increased (Bozoki et al., 2001). Neuroimaging measures have also been reported to significantly improve the predictive accuracy of cognitive instruments (Grundman et al., 2004; Visser, Verhey, Hofman et al., 2002). Therefore, convergent methods could allow the development of useful predictive algorithms which could be adopted by clinicians. Nevertheless, the proposed algorithms must be kept as parsimonious as possible in order to be applicable in multiple clinical settings (Petersen and O'Brien, 2006).

The difficulty in clearly identifying, at a preclinical dementia stage, the subsequent clinical evolution of patients may be due to the fact that the borderline zone between MCI and mild dementia is a continuum rather than a sharp boundary (Perneczky, Pohl, Sorg, Hartmann, Tosic et al., 2006). Currently, the conversion from MCI to dementia is defined in terms of dichotomous outcomes, i.e. converters versus non-converters at a precise endpoint. By doing so, it cannot rule out the hypothesis that the non-converter group may include both patients who may later develop dementia and patients who never will (Chetelat et al., 2005).

This raises the question about the validity of this definition of conversion. Therefore, it might be in vain to predict future conversion to dementia from performance on a test at a single time point. Evaluating the predictive power of change scores could be an interesting alternative (Tian, 2003).

CONCLUSION

A lot of work remains to be done regarding the definition and assessment of the possible various preclinical states of dementia. Prospective cohort validation studies including the administration of cognitive screening tests at baseline and clinicopathological correlations are still lacking. These studies are essential to determine the capacity of a screening test to predict the final diagnosis and to verify whether it can discriminate between subtypes of MCI, as prodromal stages of AD, and other dementias. However, the results of the reviewed studies on the MMSE, CAMCOG, ADAS-Cog and MDRS as well as our preliminary findings presented in this chapter indicate that some of these cognitive screening measures, particularly the MDRS and ADAS-Cog, may be useful to distinguish MCI of the amnesic type from normal aging and Alzheimer's disease, especially if they are used with convergent screening methods.

Nevertheless, one should keep in mind the danger in misinterpreting scores on a given screening measure and considering these results as a diagnostic certainty. Screening tests were not elaborated for that purpose. Unless the impairment is so important to be non equivocal, they only indicate that the patient is susceptible to be affected by the disease. This should be taken in consideration even more with MCI since not all individuals with MCI will develop dementia in the future. A single administration of a screening test gives only a measure of current cognitive functioning, and does not provide an assessment of deterioration from a previous level, which constitutes a diagnostic criterion both for dementia (e.g. DSM-IV) and MCI. Consequently, the diagnosis of dementia and MCI requires reliable independent information from an informant who has known the patient long enough before the onset of symptoms in order to observe a significant decline. Even if the MCI does not convert to dementia, the consequences for aging individuals presenting with MCI can surely be deleterious for their quality of life and self-esteem. Therefore, detecting the presence of MCI as early as possible is crucial in order to provide appropriate social support, treatment and management to elderly people.

ACKNOWLEDGEMENTS

This work was supported by the Alzheimer Society of Canada, and by the Fonds de la Recherche en Santé du Québec (doctoral awards to Evelyne Matteau).

REFERENCES

Aarsland, D., Litvan, I., Salmon, D., Galasko, D., Wentzel-Larsen, T., and Larsen, J. P. (2003). Performance on the Dementia Rating Scale in Parkinson's disease with dementia and dementia with Lewy bodies: comparison with progressive supranuclear palsy and Alzheimer's disease. *Journal of Neurology and Neurosurgery Psychiatry, 74*, 1215-1220.

Albert, M. S., Moss, M. B., Tanzi, R., and Jones, K. (2001). Preclinical prediction of AD using neuropsychological tests. *Journal of International Neuropsychology Society, 7*(5), 631-639.

Alladi, S., Arnold, R., Mitchell, J., Nestor, P. J., and Hodges, J. R. (2006). Mild cognitive impairment: applicability of research criteria in a memory clinic and characterization of cognitive profile. *Psychological Medicine, 36*(4), 507-515.

American Psychiatric Association, A. (1994). *Diagnostic and Statistical Manual of Mental Disorders* (4ième ed.). Washington, DC: American Psychiatric Association.

American Psychiatric Association, A. (1998). Guidelines for the evaluation of dementia and age-related cognitive decline. *American Psychologist, 53*, 1298-1303.

Anastasi, A., and Urbina, S. (1997). *Psychological Testing* (7th ed.). New Jersey: Prentice Hall.

Anonymous. The Canadian Study of Health and Aging: risk factors for Alzheimer's disease in Canada. *Neurology* 1994, 44, 2073-2080.

Arikuni, T., Sako, H., and Murata, A. (1994). Ipsilateral connections of the anterior cingulate cortex with the frontal and medial temporal cortices in the macaque monkey. *Neurosciences Research, 21*(1), 19-39.

Backman, L., Jones, S., Berger, A. K., Laukka, E. J., and Small, B. J. (2004). Multiple cognitive deficits during the transition to Alzheimer's disease. *Journal of Internal Medicine, 256*(3), 195-204.

Backman, L., Jones, S., Berger, A. K., Laukka, E. J., and Small, B. J. (2005). Cognitive impairment in preclinical Alzheimer's disease: a meta-analysis. *Neuropsychology, 19*(4), 520-531.

Benson, A. D., Slavin, M. J., Tran, T. T., Petrella, J. R., and Doraiswamy, P. M. (2005). Screening for Early Alzheimer's Disease: Is There Still a Role for the Mini-Mental State Examination? *Primary Care Companion Journal of Clinical Psychiatry, 7*(2), 62-69.

Blessed, G., Black, S. E., Butler, T., and Kay, D. W. (1991). The diagnosis of dementia in the elderly. A comparison of CAMCOG (the cognitive section of CAMDEX), the AGECAT program, DSM-III, the Mini-Mental State Examination and some short rating scales. *British Journal of Psychiatry, 159*, 193-198.

Boeve, B., McCormick, J., Smith, G., Ferman, T., Rummans, T., Carpenter, T., et al. (2003). Mild cognitive impairment in the oldest old. *Neurology, 60*(3), 477-480.

Bozoki, A., Giordani, B., Heidebrink, J. L., Berent, S., and Foster, N. L. (2001). Mild cognitive impairments predict dementia in nondemented elderly patients with memory loss. *Archives of Neurology, 58*(3), 411-416.

Cabranes, J. A., De Juan, R., Encinas, M., Marcos, A., Gil, P., Fernandez, C., et al. (2004). Relevance of functional neuroimaging in the progression of mild cognitive impairment. *Neurology Research, 26*(5), 496-501.

Callahan, C. M., Hendrie, H. C., and Tierney, W. M. (1995). Documentation and evaluation of cognitive impairment in elderly primary care patients. *Annals of Internal Medicine, 122*(6), 422-429.

Canadian Study of Health and Aging Working Group. (2000). The incidence of dementia in Canada. *Neurology, 55*(1), 66-73.

Chan, A. S., Choi, M. K., and Salmon, D. P. (2001). The effects of age, education, and gender on the Mattis Dementia Rating Scale performance of elderly Chinese and American individuals. *Journal of Gerontology B: Psychological Sciences and Social Sciences, 56*(6), 356-363.

Chetelat, G., Eustache, F., Viader, F., De La Sayette, V., Pelerin, A., Mezenge, F., et al. (2005). FDG-PET measurement is more accurate than neuropsychological assessments to predict global cognitive deterioration in patients with mild cognitive impairment. *Neurocase, 11*(1), 14-25.

Chong, M. S., and Sahadevan, S. (2005). Preclinical Alzheimer's disease: diagnosis and prediction of progression. *Lancet Neurology, 4*(9), 576-579.

Coblentz, J. M., Mattis, S., Zingesser, L. H., Kasoff, S. S., Wisniewski, H. M., and Katzman, R. (1973). Presenile dementia. Clinical aspects and evaluation of cerebrospinal fluid dynamics. *Archives of Neurology, 29*(5), 299-308.

Collie, A., and Maruff, P. (2000). The neuropsychology of preclinical Alzheimer's disease and mild cognitive impairment. *Neuroscience and Biobehavioral Reviews, 24*(3), 365-374.

Collie, A., and Maruff, P. (2002). An analysis of systems of classifying mild cognitive impairment in older people. *Australian and New Zealand Journal of Psychiatry, 36*(1), 133-140.

Cotter, R. B., Burke, J. D., Loeber, R., and Navratil, J. L. (2002). Innovative retention methods in longitudinal research: A case study of the developmental trends study. *Journal of Child and Family Studies, 11*, 485-498.

Crum, R. M., Anthony, J. C., Bassett, S. S., and Folstein, M. F. (1993). Population-based norms for the Mini-Mental State Examination by age and educational level. *Journal of the American Medical Association, 269*(18), 2386-2391.

Deeks, J. J., and Altman, D. G. (2004). Diagnostic Tests 4: likelihood ratios. *British Medical Journal, 329*, 168-169.

Delis, D. C., Kramer, J. H., Kaplan, E. F., and Ober, B. A. (1987). *California Verbal Learning Test: Adult Version Manual.* San Antonio, TX: The Psychological Corporation.

Demakis, G. J., Mercury, M. G., and Sweet, J. J. (2000). Screening for cognitive impairments in primary care settings. In M. E. Maruish (Ed.), *Handbook of Psychological Assessment in Primary Care Settings*, (pp. 555-582). Mahwah, NJ: Lawrence Erlbaum Associates, Inc.

Derogatis, L. R., and Lynn, L. L. (2000). Screening and monitoring psychiatric disorder in primary care populations. In M. E. Maruish (Ed.), *Handbook of Psychological Assessment in Primary Care Settings*, (pp. 115-152). Mahwah, NJ: Lawrence Erlbaum Associates, Inc.

deToledo-Morrell, L., Stoub, T. R., Bulgakova, M., Wilson, R. S., Bennett, D. A., Leurgans, S., et al. (2004). MRI-derived entorhinal volume is a good predictor of conversion from MCI to AD. *Neurobiology of Aging, 25*(9), 1197-1203.

Dickerson, B. C., Goncharova, I., Sullivan, M. P., Forchetti, C., Wilson, R. S., Bennett, D. A., et al. (2001). MRI-derived entorhinal and hippocampal atrophy in incipient and very mild Alzheimer's disease. *Neurobiology of Aging, 22*(5), 747-754.

Feldman, H. H., and Jacova, C. (2005). Mild cognitive impairment. *American Journal of Geriatric Psychiatry, 13*(8), 645-655.

Fields, R. B. (1998). The Dementias. In P. D. Nussbaum (Ed.), *Clinical Neuropsychology: A Pocket Handbook for Assessment*, (pp. 211-239). Washington: American Psychological Association.

Folstein, M. F., Folstein, S. E., and McHugh, P. R. (1975). "Mini-mental state". A practical method for grading the cognitive state of patients for the clinician. *Journal of Psychiatric Research, 12*(3), 189-198.

Fountoulakis, K. N., Tsolakis, M., and Kazis, A. (2001). Investigation of «borderline» dementia, particularly of Alzheimer's type, compared with non-demented patients with similar neuropsychological profiles. *International Journal of Psychiatry in Clinical Practice, 5*, 55-61.

Franzen, M. D. (2000). *Reliability and Validity in Neuropsychological Assessment* (2nd ed.). New York: Kluwer Academic/Plenum Publishers.

Freidl, W., Stronegger, W. J., Berghold, A., Reinhart, B., Petrovic, K., and Schmidt, R. (2002). The agreement of the Mattis Dementia Rating Scale with the Mini-Mental State Examination. *International Journal of Geriatric Psychiatry, 17*(7), 685-686.

Galasko, D., Bennett, D., Sano, M., Ernesto, C., Thomas, R., Grundman, M., et al. (1997). An inventory to assess activities of daily living for clinical trials in Alzheimer's disease. The Alzheimer's Disease Cooperative Study. *Alzheimer Disease and Associated Disorders, 11 Suppl 2*, S33-39.

Ganguli, M., Dodge, H. H., Shen, C., and DeKosky, S. T. (2004). Mild cognitive impairment, amnestic type: an epidemiologic study. *Neurology, 63*(1), 115-121.

Ganguli, M., Rodriguez, E., Mulsant, B., Richards, S., Pandav, R., Bilt, J. V., et al. (2004). Detection and management of cognitive impairment in primary care: The Steel Valley Seniors Survey. *Journal of American Geriatric Society, 52*(10), 1668-1675.

Geslani, D. M., Tierney, M. C., Herrmann, N., and Szalai, J. P. (2005). Mild cognitive impairment: an operational definition and its conversion rate to Alzheimer's disease. *Dementia and Geriatric Cognitive Disorders, 19*(5-6), 383-389.

Gifford, D. R., and Cummings, J. L. (1999). Evaluating dementia screening tests: methodologic standards to rate their performance. *Neurology, 52*(2), 224-227.

Gomez-Isla, T., Price, J. L., McKeel, D. W., Jr., Morris, J. C., Growdon, J. H., and Hyman, B. T. (1996). Profound loss of layer II entorhinal cortex neurons occurs in very mild Alzheimer's disease. *Journal of Neurosciences, 16*(14), 4491-4500.

Grady, C. L., Haxby, J. V., Horwitz, B., Sundaram, M., Berg, G., Schapiro, M., et al. (1988). Longitudinal study of the early neuropsychological and cerebral metabolic changes in dementia of the Alzheimer type. *Journal of Clinical and Experimental Neuropsychology, 10*(5), 576-596.

Graham, D. P., Cully, J. A., Snow, A. L., Massman, P., and Doody, R. (2004). The Alzheimer's Disease Assessment Scale-Cognitive subscale: normative data for older adult controls. *Alzheimer's Disease and Associated Disorders, 18*(4), 236-240.

Graham, J. E., Rockwood, K., Beattie, B. L., Eastwood, R., Gauthier, S., Tuokko, H., et al. (1997). Prevalence and severity of cognitive impairment with and without dementia in an elderly population. *Lancet, 349*(9068), 1793-1796.

Green, R. C., Woodard, J. L., and Green, J. (1995). Validity of the Mattis Dementia Rating Scale for detection of cognitive impairment in the elderly. *Journal of Neuropsychiatry and Clinical Neurosciences, 7*(3), 357-360.

Griffith, H. R., Netson, K. L., Harrell, L. E., Zamrini, E. Y., Brockington, J. C., and Marson, D. C. (2006). Amnestic mild cognitive impairment: diagnostic outcomes and clinical prediction over a two-year time period. *Journal of the International Neuropsychological Society, 12*(2), 166-175.

Grundman, M., Petersen, R. C., Ferris, S. H., Thomas, R. G., Aisen, P. S., Bennett, D. A., et al. (2004). Mild cognitive impairment can be distinguished from Alzheimer disease and normal aging for clinical trials. *Archives of Neurology, 61*(1), 59-66.

Hebert, L. E., Scherr, P. A., Bienias, J. L., Bennett, D. A., and Evans, D. A. (2003). Alzheimer disease in the US population: prevalence estimates using the 2000 census. *Archives of Neurology, 60*(8), 1119-1122.

Hodges, J. R., Erzinclioglu, S., and Patterson, K. (2006). Evolution of cognitive deficits and conversion to dementia in patients with mild cognitive impairment: a very-long-term follow-up study. *Dementia and Geriatric Cognitive Disorders, 21*(5-6), 380-391.

Hohl, U., Grundman, M., Salmon, D. P., Thomas, R. G., and Thal, L. J. (1999). Mini-Mental State Examination and Mattis Dementia Rating Scale performance differs in Hispanic and non-Hispanic Alzheimer's disease patients. *Journal of International Neuropsychology Society, 5*(4), 301-307.

Hughes, C. P., Berg, L., Danziger, W. L., Coben, L. A., and Martin, R. L. (1982). A new clinical scale for the staging of dementia. *British Journal of Psychiatry, 140*, 566-572.

Huppert, F. A., Jorm, A. F., Brayne, C., Girling, D. M., Barkley, C., Beardsall, L., et al. (1996). Psychometric properties of the CAMCOG and its efficacy in the diagnosis of dementia. *Aging, Neuropsychology, and Cognition, 3*(3), 201-214.

Isella, V., Villa, L., Russo, A., Regazzoni, R., Ferrarese, C., and Appollonio, I. M. (2006). Discriminative and predictive power of an informant report in mild cognitive impairment. *Journal of Neurology and Neurosurgery Psychiatry, 77*(2), 166-171.

Jackson, M. D., and Ramsdell, J. W. (1988). Use of the Mini-Mental State Examination (MMSE) to screen for dementia in elderly outpatients. *Journal of American Geriatric Society, 36*, 662.

Jaeschke, R., Guyatt, G., and Lijmer, J. (2002). Diagnostic tests. In G. Guyatt and D. Rennie (Eds.), *User's guides to the medical literature*, (pp. 121-140). Chicago: American Medical Association Press.

Jean, L., Simard, M., Van Reekum, R., and Clarke, D. E. (2005). Differential cognitive impairment in subjects with geriatric depression who will develop Alzheimer's disease and other dementias: A retrospective study. *International Psychogeriatrics, 17*, 289-301.

Jelle Visser, P., Verhey, F. R., Jolles, J., and Jonker, C. (2002). Course of minimal dementia and predictors of outcome. *International Journal of Geriatric Psychiatry, 17*(9), 835-841.

Jorm, A. F., and Korten, A. E. (1988). Assessment of cognitive decline in the elderly by informant interview. *British Journal of Psychiatry, 152*, 209-213.

Kazdin, A. E. (2003). *Research Design in Clinical Psychology* (Fourth ed.). Boston: Allyn and Bacon.

Kobak, K. A., Mundt, J. C., and Katzelnick, D. J. (2000). Future directions in psychological assessment and treatment in primary care settings. In M. E. Maruish (Ed.), *Handbook of Psychological Assessment in Primary Care Settings*, (pp. 763-796). Mahwah, NJ: Lawrence Erlbaum Associates, Inc.

Kokmen, E., Naessens, J. M., and Offord, K. P. (1987). A short test of mental status: description and preliminary results. *Mayo Clinic Proceedings, 62*(4), 281-288.

Lam, L. C. W., Lui, V. W. C., Chiu, H. F. K., and Chan, S. S. M. (2005). Executive function impairment in community elderly subjects with questionable dementia. *Dementia and Geriatric Cognitive Disorders, 19*, 86-90.

Lam, L. C. W., Lui, V. W. C., Chiu, H. F. K., and Chan, S. S. M. (2006). Executive function impairment in community elderly subjects with questionable dementia. *Dementia and Geriatric Cognitive Disorders, 19*, 86-90.

Larrieu, S., Letenneur, L., Orgogozo, J. M., Fabrigoule, C., Amieva, H., Le Carret, N., et al. (2002). Incidence and outcome of mild cognitive impairment in a population-based prospective cohort. *Neurology, 59*(10), 1594-1599.

Lee, D. Y., Youn, J. C., Choo, I. H., Kim, K. W., Jhoo, J. H., Pak, Y. S., et al. (2006). Combination of clinical and neuropsychologic information as a better predictor of the progression to Alzheimer disease in questionable dementia individuals. *American Journal of Geriatric Psychiatry, 14*(2), 130-138.

Lehrner, J., Gufler, R., Guttmann, G., Maly, J., Gleiss, A., Auff, E., et al. (2005). Annual conversion to alzheimer disease among patients with memory complaints attending an outpatient memory clinic: the influence of amnestic mild cognitive impairment and the predictive value of neuropsychological testing. *Wiener Klinische Wochenschrift, 117*(18), 629-635.

Lezak, M. D. (1995). *Neuropsychological Assessment* (3rd ed.). New York: Oxford University Press.

Lezak, M. D., Howieson, D. B., and Loring, D. W. (2004). *Neuropsychological Assessment* (4th ed.). New York: Oxford University Press.

Li, M., Ng, T. P., Kua, E. H., and Ko, S. M. (2006). Brief informant screening test for mild cognitive impairment and early Alzheimer's disease. *Dementia and Geriatric Cognitive Disorders, 21*(5-6), 392-402.

Lindeboom, J., Ter Horst, R., Hooyer, C., Dinkgreve, M., and Jonker, C. (1993). Some psychometric properties of the CAMCOG. *Psychological Medicine, 23*(1), 213-219.

Lolk, A., Nielsen, H., Andersen, K., Andersen, J., and Kragh-Sorensen, P. (2000). CAMCOG as a screening instrument for dementia: the Odense study. Cambridge Cognitive Examination. *Acta Psychiatrica Scandinavica, 102*(5), 331-335.

Lopez, O. L., Jagust, W. J., DeKosky, S. T., Becker, J. T., Fitzpatrick, A., Dulberg, C., et al. (2003). Prevalence and classification of mild cognitive impairment in the Cardiovascular Health Study Cognition Study: part 1. *Archives of Neurology, 60*(10), 1385-1389.

Lucas, J. A., Ivnik, R. J., Smith, G. E., Bohac, D. L., Tangalos, E. G., Kokmen, E., et al. (1998). Normative data for the Mattis Dementia Rating Scale. *Journal of Clinical and Experimental Neuropsychology, 20*(4), 536-547.

Luis, C. A., Loewenstein, D. A., Acevedo, A., Barker, W. W., and Duara, R. (2003). Mild cognitive impairment: directions for future research. *Neurology, 61*(4), 438-444.

Marcopulos, B. A., McLain, C. A., and Giuliano, A. J. (1997). Cognitive impairment or inadequate norms: A study of healthy, rural older adults with limited education. *The Clinical Neuropsychologist, 11*, 111-131.

Mattis, S. (1976). Mental Status Examination for organic mental syndrome in the elderly patient. In L. Bellak and T. B. Karasu (Eds.), *Geriatric Psychiatry: A handbook for psychiatrists and primary care physicians*, (pp. 77-121). New York: Grune and Stratton.

McDowell, I., Kristjansson, B., Hill, G. B., and Hebert, R. (1997). Community screening for dementia: the Mini Mental State Exam (MMSE) and Modified Mini-Mental State Exam (3MS) compared. *Journal of Clinical Epidemiology, 50*(4), 377-383.

McKhann, G., Drachman, D., Folstein, M., Katzman, R., Price, D., and Stadlan, E. M. (1984). Clinical diagnosis of Alzheimer's disease: Report of the NINCDS-ADRDA Work Group under the auspices of Department of Health and Human, Services Task Force on Alzheimer's disease. *Neurology, 34*, 939-944.

Meiran, N., Stuss, D. T., Guzman, D. A., Lafleche, G., and Willmer, J. (1996). Diagnosis of dementia. Methods for interpretation of scores of five neuropsychological tests. *Archives of Neurology, 53*(10), 1043-1054.

Milberg, W. (1996). Issues in the Assessment of cognitive function in dementia. *Brain and Cognition, 31*, 114-132.

Monsch, A. U., Bondi, M. W., Salmon, D. P., Butters, N., Thal, L. J., Hansen, L. A., et al. (1995). Clinical validity of the Mattis Dementia Rating Scale in detecting Dementia of the Alzheimer type. A double cross-validation and application to a community-dwelling sample. *Archives of Neurology, 52*(9), 899-904.

Morris, J. C. (1993). The Clinical Dementia Rating (CDR): current version and scoring rules. *Neurology, 43*(11), 2412-2414.

Morris, J. C., Storandt, M., Miller, J. P., McKeel, D. W., Price, J. L., Rubin, E. H., et al. (2001). Mild cognitive impairment represents early-stage Alzheimer disease. *Archives of Neurology, 58*(3), 397-405.

Morris, R. G., and Becker, J. T. (Eds.). (2004). *Cognitive Neuropsychology of Alzheimer's Disease* (2nd ed.). New York: Oxford University Press.

Morris, R. G., and James, T. B. (2004). A Cognitive Neuropsychology of Alzheimer's Disease. In R. G. Morris and T. B. James (Eds.), *Cognitive Neuropsychology of Alzheimer's Disease*, 2nd ed., (pp. 3-8). New York: Oxford University Press.

Mosconi, L., Perani, D., Sorbi, S., Herholz, K., Nacmias, B., Holthoff, V., et al. (2004). MCI conversion to dementia and the APOE genotype: a prediction study with FDG-PET. *Neurology, 63*(12), 2332-2340.

Nelson, A., Fogel, B. S., and Faust, D. (1986). Bedside cognitive screening instruments. A critical assessment. *Journal of Nervous and Mental Disorders, 174*(2), 73-83.

Nestor, P. J., Scheltens, P., and Hodges, J. R. (2004). Advances in the early detection of Alzheimer's disease. *National Medicine, 10 Suppl*, S34-41.

Panza, F., D'Introno, A., Colacicco, A. M., Capurso, C., Del Parigi, A., Caselli, R. J., et al. (2005). Current epidemiology of mild cognitive impairment and other predementia syndromes. *American Journal of Geriatric Psychiatry, 13*(8), 633-644.

Paolo, A. M., Troster, A. I., Glatt, S. L., Hubble, J. P., and Koller, W. C. (1995). Differentiation of the dementias of Alzheimer's and Parkinson's disease with the Dementia Rating Scale. *Journal of Geriatric Psychiatry and Neurology, 8*(3), 184-188.

Patterson, C., Gauthier, S., Bergman, H., Cohen, C., Feightner, J. W., Feldman, H., et al. (2001). The recognition, assessment and management of dementing disorders: conclusions from the Canadian Consensus Conference on Dementia. *Canadian Journal of Neurological Sciences, 28 Suppl 1*, S3-16.

Paulsen, J. S., Butters, N., Sadek, J. R., Johnson, S. A., Salmon, D. P., Swerdlow, N. R., et al. (1995). Distinct cognitive profiles of cortical and subcortical dementia in advanced illness. *Neurology, 45*(5), 951-956.

Perneczky, R., Pohl, C., Sorg, C., Hartmann, J., Komossa, K., Alexopoulos, P., et al. (2006). Complex activities of daily living in mild cognitive impairment: conceptual and diagnostic issues. *Age and Ageing, 35*(3), 240-245.

Perneczky, R., Pohl, C., Sorg, C., Hartmann, J., Tosic, N., Grimmer, T., et al. (2006). Impairment of activities of daily living requiring memory or complex reasoning as part of the MCI syndrome. *International Journal of Geriatric Psychiatry, 21*(2), 158-162.

Petersen, R. C. (2004). Mild cognitive impairment as a diagnostic entity. *Journal of Internal Medicine, 256*(3), 183-194.

Petersen, R. C., and O'Brien, J. (2006). Mild cognitive impairment should be considered for DSM-V. *Journal of Geriatric Psychiatry and Neurology, 19*(3), 147-154.

Petersen, R. C., Smith, G. E., Waring, S. C., Ivnik, R. J., Tangalos, E. G., and Kokmen, E. (1999). Mild Cognitive Impairment: Clinical Characterization and Outcome. *Archives of Neurology, 56*, 303-308.

Petersen, R. C., Stevens, J. C., Ganguli, M., Tangalos, E. G., Cummings, J. L., and DeKosky, S. T. (2001). Practice parameter: early detection of dementia: mild cognitive impairment (an evidence-based review). Report of the Quality Standards Subcommittee of the American Academy of Neurology. *Neurology, 56*(9), 1133-1142.

Petersen, R. C., and Morris, J. C. (2003). Clinical Features. In R. C. Peterson (Ed.), *Mild Cognitive Impairment: Aging to Alzheimer's Disease*, (pp. 15-39). New York: Oxford University Press.

Post, S. G. (1999). Future scenarios for the prevention and delay of Alzheimer disease onset in high-risk groups. An ethical perspective. *American Journal of Preventive Medicine, 16*(2), 105-110.

Pyo, G., Elble, R. J., Ala, T., and Markwell, S. J. (2006). The characteristics of patients with uncertain/mild cognitive impairment on the Alzheimer disease assessment scale-cognitive subscale. *Alzheimer Disease and Associated Disorders, 20*(1), 16-22.

Rascovsky, K., Salmon, D. P., Ho, G. J., Galasko, D., Peavy, G. M., Hansen, L. A., et al. (2002). Cognitive profiles differ in autopsy-confirmed frontotemporal dementia and AD. *Neurology, 58*(12), 1801-1808.

Ravaglia, G., Forti, P., Maioli, F., Servadei, L., Martelli, M., Brunetti, N., et al. (2005). Screening for mild cognitive impairment in elderly ambulatory patients with cognitive complaints. *Aging of Clinical and Experimental Research, 17*(5), 374-379.

Rey, A. (1958). *Mémorisation d'une série de 15 mots en 5 répétitions*. Paris: Presse Universitaire de France.

Rosen, W. G., Mohs, R. C., and Davis, K. L. (1984). A new rating scale for Alzheimer's disease. *American Journal of Psychiatry, 141*(11), 1356-1364.

Rosser, A. E., and Hodges, J. R. (1994). The Dementia Rating Scale in Alzheimer's disease, Huntington's disease and progressive supranuclear palsy. *Journal of Neurology, 241*(9), 531-536.

Roth, M., Tym, E., Mountjoy, C. Q., Huppert, F. A., Hendrie, H., Verma, S., et al. (1986). CAMDEX. A standardised instrument for the diagnosis of mental disorder in the elderly with special reference to the early detection of dementia. *British Journal of Psychiatry, 149*, 698-709.

Rublìk, F. (2001). On performance of multiple comparison methods used in conjunction with the Kruskal-Wallis test. *Measurement Science Review, 1*(1), 37-42.

Sackett, D. L., Straus, S., Richardson, W. S., Rosenberg, W., and Haynes, R. B. (2000). *Evidence-based medicine. How to practise and teach EBM.* (2nd ed.). Edinburgh: Churchill Livingstone.

Salmon, D. D., Kwo-on-Yuen, P. F., Heindel, W. C., Butters, N., and Thal, L. J. (1989). Differentiation of Alzheimer's disease and Huntington's disease with the Dementia Rating Scale. *Archives of Neurology, 36*, 1204-1208.

Salmon, D. P., Thal, L. J., Butters, N., and Heindel, W. C. (1990). Longitudinal evaluation of dementia of the Alzheimer type: a comparison of three standardized mental status examinations. *Neurology, 40*(8), 1225-1230.

Schmidt, K. S., Mattis, P. J., Adams, J., and Nestor, P. (2005a). Alternate-form reliability of the Dementia Rating Scale-2. *Archives of Clinical Neuropsychology, 20*(4), 435-441.

Schmidt, K. S., Mattis, P. J., Adams, J., and Nestor, P. (2005b). Test-Retest Reliability of the Dementia Rating Scale-2: Alternate Form. *Dementia and Geriatric Cognitive Disorders, 20*(1), 42-44.

Schmidt, R., Freidl, W., Fazekas, F., Reinhart, B., Grieshofer, P., Koch, M., et al. (1994). The Mattis Dementia Rating Scale: normative data from 1,001 healthy volunteers. *Neurology, 44*(5), 964-966.

Simard, M.. (1998). Mini-Mental-State-Examination: Strengths and Weaknesses of a Cognitive Instrument. *Canadian Alzheimer's Disease Review, 2*(3), 10-12.

Simard, M., and Sampson, E.L. (In press). Dementia: Pharmacological and Non-Pharmacological Treatments and Guideline Review. In P. Tyrer and K. Silk (Eds.), *The Cambridge Textbook of Effective Treatment in Psychiatry.*). Cambridge: Cambridge University Press.

Simard, M., and van Reekum, R. (1999). Memory assessment in studies of cognition-enhancing drugs for Alzheimer's disease. *Drugs and Aging, 14*(3), 197-230.

Simard, M., Van Reekum, R., and Suvajac, B. (2000). Improving cognition, behavior, and function, and slowing disease progression of Alzheimer's disease. *Clinical Geriatrics, 8*(11), 32-58.

Smith, G. E., Ivnik, R. J., Malec, J. F., Kokmen, E., Tangalos, E., and Petersen, R. C. (1994). Psychometric Properties of the Mattis Dementia Rating Scale. *Assessment, 1*(2), 123-132.

Spreen, O., and Strauss, E. (1998). *A Compendium of Neurosychological Tests: Administration, Norms, and Commentary* (2nd ed.). New York, NY: Oxford University Press, Inc.

Strauss, E., Sherman, E. M., and Spreen, O. (2006). *A compendium of neuropsychological tests: Administration, Norms, and Commentary* (3rd ed.). New York: Oxford University Press.

Streiner, D. L. (2002). The case of the missing data: methods of dealing with dropouts and other research vagaries. *Canadian Journal of Psychiatry, 47*(1), 68-75.

Stuss, D. T., Meiran, N., Guzman, D. A., Lafleche, G., and Willmer, J. (1996). Do long tests yield a more accurate diagnosis of dementia than short tests? A comparison of five neuropsychological tests. *Archives of Neurology, 53*(10), 1033-1039.

Tabert, M. H., Albert, S. M., Borukhova-Milov, L., Camacho, Y., Pelton, G., Liu, X., et al. (2002). Functional deficits in patients with mild cognitive impairment: prediction of AD. *Neurology, 58*(5), 758-764.

Tabert, M. H., Manly, J. J., Liu, X., Pelton, G. H., Rosenblum, S., Jacobs, M., et al. (2006). Neuropsychological prediction of conversion to Alzheimer disease in patients with mild cognitive impairment. *Archives of General Psychiatry, 63*(8), 916-924.

Tangalos, E. G., Smith, G. E., Ivnik, R. J., Petersen, R. C., Kokmen, E., Kurland, L. T., et al. (1996). The Mini-Mental State Examination in general medical practice: clinical utility and acceptance. *Mayo Clinic Proceedings, 71*(9), 829-837.

Tang-Wai, D. F., Knopman, D. S., Geda, Y. E., Edland, S. D., Smith, G. E., Ivnik, R. J., et al. (2003). Comparison of the short test of mental status and the mini-mental state examination in mild cognitive impairment. *Archives of Neurology, 60*(12), 1777-1781.

Tian, J., Bucks, R. S., Haworth, J., and Wilcock, G. (2003). Neuropsychological prediction of conversion to dementia from questionable dementia: statistically significant but not yet clinically useful. *Journal of Neurology and Neurosurgery Psychiatry, 74*(4), 433-438.

Tierney, M. C., Herrmann, N., Geslani, D. M., and Szalai, J. P. (2003). Contribution of informant and patient ratings to the accuracy of the mini-mental state examination in predicting probable Alzheimer's disease. *Journal of American Geriatric Society, 51*(6), 813-818.

Tombaugh, T. N., McDowell, I., Kristjansson, B., and Hubley, A. M. (1996). Mini-Mental State Examination (MMSE) and the Modified MMSE (3MS): A psychometric comparison and normative data. *Psychological Assessment, 8*, 48-59.

Tombaugh, T. N., and McIntyre, N. J. (1992). The mini-mental state examination: a comprehensive review. *Journal of American and Geriatric Society, 40*(9), 922-935.

van der Flier, W. M., van der Vlies, A. E., Weverling-Rijnsburger, A. W., de Boer, N. L., Admiraal-Behloul, F., Bollen, E. L., et al. (2005). MRI measures and progression of cognitive decline in nondemented elderly attending a memory clinic. *International Journal of Geriatric Psychiatry, 20*(11), 1060-1066.

Vangel, S. J., and Lichtenberg, P. A. (1995). Mattis Dementia Rating Scale: Clinical Utility and relationship with demographic variables. *The Clinical Neuropsychologist, 9*, 209-213.

Visser, P. J., Verhey, F. R., Hofman, P. A., Scheltens, P., and Jolles, J. (2002). Medial temporal lobe atrophy predicts Alzheimer's disease in patients with minor cognitive impairment. *Journal of Neurology and Neurosurgery Psychiatry, 72*(4), 491-497.

Visser, P. J., Verhey, F. R., Jolles, J., and Jonker, C. (2002). Course of minimal dementia and predictors of outcome. *International Journal of Geriatric Psychiatry, 17*(9), 835-841.

Visser, P. J., Verhey, F. R., Ponds, R. W., and Jolles, J. (2001). Diagnosis of preclinical Alzheimer's disease in a clinical setting. *International Psychogeriatrics, 13*(4), 411-423.

Vitaliano, P. P., Breen, A. R., Russo, J., Albert, M., Vitiello, M. V., and Prinz, P. N. (1984). The clinical utility of the Dementia Rating Scale for assessing Alzheimer patients. *Journal of Chronic Disorders, 37*(9-10), 743-753.

Wang, Q. S., and Zhou, J. N. (2002). Retrieval and encoding of episodic memory in normal aging and patients with mild cognitive impairment. *Brain Research*, 924(1), 113-115.

Warner, J. (2004). Clinicians' guide to evaluating diagnostic and screening tests in psychiatry. *Advances in Psychiatric Treatment*, 10, 446-454.

Williams, J. G., Huppert, F. A., Matthews, F. E., and Nickson, J. (2003). Performance and normative values of a concise neuropsychological test (CAMCOG) in an elderly population sample. *International Journal of Geriatric Psychiatry*, 18(7), 631-644.

Wolf, H., Grunwald, M., Ecke, G. M., Zedlick, D., Bettin, S., Dannenberg, C., et al. (1998). The prognosis of mild cognitive impairment in the elderly. *Journal of Neural Transmission,* Suppl. 54, 31-50.

Woodard, J. L., Auchus, A. P., Godsall, R. E., and Green, R. C. (1998). An analysis of test bias and differential item functioning due to race on the Mattis Dementia Rating Scale. *Journal of Gerontology B: Psychological Sciences and Social Sciences*, 53(6), 370-374.

Xu, G., Meyer, J. S., Thornby, J., Chowdhury, M., and Quach, M. (2002). Screening for mild cognitive impairment (MCI) utilizing combined mini-mental-cognitive capacity examinations for identifying dementia prodromes. *International Journal of Geriatric Psychiatry*, 17(11), 1027-1033.

Yesavage, J. A., O'Hara, R., Kraemer, H., Noda, A., Taylor, J. L., Ferris, S., et al. (2002). Modeling the prevalence and incidence of Alzheimer's disease and mild cognitive impairment. *Journal of Psychiatric Research*, 36(5), 281-286.

Zec, R. F., Landreth, E. S., Vicari, S. K., Feldman, E., Belman, J., Andrise, A., et al. (1992). Alzheimer disease assessment scale: useful for both early detection and staging of dementia of the Alzheimer type. *Alzheimer Disease and Associated Disorders*, 6(2), 89-102.

In: Leading-Edge Cognitive Disorders Research
Editor: James P. Tsai, pp. 59-63
ISBN: 978-1-60021-843-9

Chapter 2

ESSENTIAL FATTY ACIDS AND COGNITION

Shlomo Yehuda, Sharon Rabinovitz and David I. Mostofsky
Psychopharmacology Laboratory,
Dept. of Psychology and Gonda Brain Research Center,
Bar Ilan University, Ramat Gan, Israel
Department of Psychology, Boston University, Boston, MA, USA

ABSTRACT

We propose that the mode of action of polyunsaturated essential fatty acids (PUFA) results from its effect in stabilizing and protecting the structure and functions of the neuronal membrane. PUFA's many effects include brain physiology that modulate pain, thermoregulation and sleep, and brain biochemistry that affects brain neurotransmitters, cholesterol, myelin, and cortisone. Related CNS disorders include Alzheimer's dementia, epilepsy and multiple sclerosis, which are notable for the disruption of normal cognitive behaviors. We further propose that not only will a deficiency in brain PUFA will lead to cognitive deficits, but that supplementation of PUFA can rehabilitate many of the consequent deficits. In addition, we conclude that the *ratio* of the two types of PUFA, viz. omega-3 and omega-6 with an optimum ratio of 1:4, is in fact even more important than the absolute level of either.

NEURONAL MEMBRANE AND PUFA

The activity of the brain is highly dependent on the integrity of the neuronal membrane. The neuronal membrane is composed mainly of proteins and lipids. The proteins in the membrane are relative stable, while the lipids exhibit a fast turnover rate. Also, it should be remembered that the neuronal membrane, the myelin sheath, surrounds the membrane, and that the myelin is composed mainly of lipids.

The physical state of the neuronal membrane is critical for the neuronal functions. The ideal state is a gel state. There are known molecules that are able to change the physical state of the membrane, for example, alcohol fluidizes the membrane, while cholesterol hardens the membrane. The change in the physical state of the neuronal membrane modifies some of the membrane functions, including neuronal information along the axon and neuronal information in the synapse.

TYPES OF PUFA

While the brain utilizes linoleic (omega-6) and alpha-linolenic (omega-3) acids *per se* for many functions, their derivatives, i.e. the longer chains of PUFA, are also important for many brain functions. It should be noted that the same enzymes that are responsible for the elongation of the fatty acids act upon both families of PUFA and compete with each other. Numerous studies have confirmed that that the level of PUFA in the neuronal membrane is very important, and recent studies have shown that the types of PUFA, and also that the ratio between omega-3 and omega-6 PUFA is just as important. For example, the ratio between the total PUFA and cholesterol level in the membrane determines the "membrane fluidity index". Not all ratios of PUFA are more equally effective in decreasing the level of cholesterol in the membrane. The ratio of 1:4 (omega-3 to omega-6) was found to be the most effective in decreasing cholesterol level in the membrane.

Consequences of Omega-3 Deficiency

The investigation of omega-3 role in various brain functions is greatly facilitated by a diet-induced deficiency. Studies have shown that omega-3 deficient rats exhibit poor learning and memory in a variety of tasks, including but not limited to Morris Water Maze performance and olfactory-based learning in addition to sensory deficits such as selected visual functions. Omega-3 deficiency induces a significant decrease in the neuron size in the hippocampus, hypothalamus and cortex; brain areas that mediate spatial and serial learning. In addition, omega-3 deficiency induces a significant reduction in cerebral catecholamines, in glucose transport capacity and glucose utilization in the brain, and in the rate of myelization. Each of these variables can be responsible for learning deficits.

Neuronal PUFA and Cognition: Animal Studies

Clearly, the various fatty acids serve different roles in the nervous system and throughout the body machinery. It has been suggested that the nervous system has an absolute molecular species requirement for proper function. Studies in our laboratory confirm this finding, and even suggest an added qualifying requirement, viz. the need for a proper ratio between the essential fatty acids. Many studies examined the effects of various fatty acids on learning and memory, but very few examined the *ratio* between various PUFA. We tested a wide range of PUFA ratios, and found that a mixture of linoleic (omega-6) and alpha-linolenic acids (omega-3) with a ratio of 4:1 was the most effective in improving learning performance (as assessed by the Morris Water Maze, and passive avoidance), elevating pain threshold, improving sleep, and improving thermoregulation. This ratio was also able to correct learning deficits induced by the neurotoxins AF64A and 5,7-dihydroxytryptamine and by 6-OH-DA (i.e. reduction in brain dopamine level).

Table 1. Effects of SR-3 on learning, physiology, CNS disorders and brain chemistry

	Dependent variable	Pretreatment	Assessment Index	Result
1. Learning	Spatial learning	(a) normal rats	Morris water tank	Reduced trials to criterion
		(b)cholinergic and serotonergic toxins; 3-weeks SR-3 treatment		Restoration of learning
		(C) EAE rats		Improvement; no complete restoration
	Passive avoidance	EAE toxin	Shock in bright/dark compartment	Repair behavior deficit
2. Physiology	Motor activity	(a) normal rats	Open field horizontal crossings and rearing	No change
		(B) EAE rats		Improvement
	Pain threshold		Hot plate/paw lick	Increased lick latency (elevated threshold)
	Thermoregul ation	IP *d*-amphetamine	Colonic temp in 4^0 C water bath	+ protection against induced hypothermia
3. CNS Disorders	Seizure threshold	SR-3	Latency and seizure stage following single convulsant dose PTZ; repeated subconvulsant doses PTZ; intraventricular $FeCl_3$; *p*-cresol sensitization to audiogenic sz.	Increased latency to major motor sz; reduced sz.duration ;
	Alzheimer dementia	SR-3	Mood; cooperation; sleep; ST memory	Improved QOL for pt and caregiver
	Multiple Sclerosis	EAE rats	Behavior	Improved
	Sleep disturbances	Human/rats	Sleep profile	Improved
4. Brain Biochemistry	Cholesterol	SR-3	Frontal cortex synaptosome analysis	Reduction in cholesterol and increase in brain EFA
	Myelin	EAE rats/ old rats		Rehabilitation of myelin
	Cortisol/ corticosteron	stress	Level of cortisol	Decrease in elevated level of stress hormones

Neuronal PUFA and Cognition: Human Studies

The results of the animal studies encouraged extensions of this research program to human studies. Several Alzheimer patients were treated with doses of the specific 1:4 mixture of PUFA. The results showed modest improvement in the Mini-Mental test, but more importantly, they showed a significant improvement in the Daily Life Questioner. Their memory improved, they could talk better, they slept better, and had fewer hallucinations. When administered to healthy subjects, the PUFA lead to reports of elevated mood, better sleep, and less prone to fatigue.

CNS Disorders and the Omega-3/Omega-6 Mixture

Our studies in animal models were not limited to an examination of memory disorders. The PUFA mixture was also found to improve the status of an experimental rat model of multiple sclerosis and a decrease in the frequency of seizures in PTZ treated rats. In addition, the compound was very effective in decreasing elevated cortisol levels in an experimental model of stress (see table 1).

Conclusion

In conclusion, the results of our studies demonstrate that essential fatty acids play a pivotal role in mediating complex processes of cognitive functions, learning and memory. In addition, the results emphasize the importance of ratio between n-3 and n-6 fatty acids. Viewing essential fatty acids as mediators of key components enables us to better understand the neuronal basis of learning and memory. While the important role of essential fatty acids is now unfolding, more studies are needed to understand the role of the individual fatty acids and comparing the profile of fatty acids in the brain and in the serum for various conditions.

References

Rabinovitz, S., Mostofsky, D.I. and Yehuda, S. (2004). Anticonvulsant efficiency, behavioral performance and cortisol level: A comparison of Carbamazepine (CBZ) and a fatty acid compound (SR-3). *Psychoneuroendocrinology, 29*, 113-124.

Yehuda, S. (2003), Omega-6/omega-3 ratio and brain related functions. In: Simopoulos, A.P and Cleland, L.G. (Eds.) *Omega-6/Omega-3 Essential Fatty Acid Ratio: The Scientific Evidence*, Karger, Basel, pp. 37-56.

Yehuda, S. and Carasso, R. L. (1993) Modulation of learning, pain thresholds, and thermoregulation in the rat by preparations of free purified α- linolenic and linoleic acids: determination of optimal n-3 to n-6 ratio. *Proc. Natl. Acad. Sci. USA, 90,* 10345-10349.

Yehuda, S., Rabinovitz S. and Mostofsky, D.I. (1999) Essential fatty acids are mediators of brain biochemistry and cognitive functions. *J. Neurosci.Res., 56,* 565-570.

Yehuda, S., Rabinovitz, S., Carasso, R.L. and Mostofsky, D. T. (2002) The Role of PUFA in aging neuronal membrane. *Neurobiology of Aging, 23*, 845-855.

In: Leading-Edge Cognitive Disorders Research
Editor: James P. Tsai, pp. 65-97
ISBN: 978-1-60021-843-9

Chapter 3

MOLECULAR BASIS OF CNS AGING, FRAILTY, FITNESS AND LONGEVITY: A MODEL BASED ON CELLULAR ENERGETICS

Kenneth G Manton [1], ***Hai Huang and Xiliang Gu***

Center for Demographic Studies, Duke University, 2117 Campus Drive, Box 90408, Durham, NC 27708, USA

ABSTRACT

The concept of frailty, a decrease in physical function and increasing vulnerability to morbidity and death, is central to the biological study of aging (Fried et al., 2001; Walston, 2004). Genetics, epigenetics, free radicals, aging, disease, and cellular bioenergetics have all been identified as causative elements in frailty. Study of these elements, and their relations, may allow us to develop dynamic models of the age related emergence of physical frailty at the population level (Dirks et al., 2006). A phenotype has been defined for physical frailty (Fried et al., 2001). An area where frailty is less completely studied is the central nervous system (CNS) where a phenotype has not been developed for cognitive "frailty". We attempt to develop such a model by examining the effects of loss of neuronal energetic capacity with age.

To develop a model of frailty in the CNS the ability to parametrically describe changes in neuronal frailty and mortality must be examined in the context of the properties of cellular processes involved in energy production. Processes whose contribution to CNS frailty are to be examined include a) shortening of the telomere by oxidative stress, b) cellular bioenergetics involving mitochondrial enzyme, membrane and matrix structure, c) select genes silencing the expression of specific proteins, and d) genomic and non-genomic thyroid hormone (*Triiodothyronine (T3))* regulation of mitochondrial structure and function, genesis and cell growth and differentiation. The role of environmental stressors, such as ionizing radiation (IR), in modifying certain rate parameters of cellular bioenergetics may suggests ways to better study and describe such mechanisms in humans.

---

[1] Corresponding author. Tel.: 919-668-2719; fax: 919-684-3861. Email address: kgm@cds.duke.edu (K.G. Manton).

I. Introduction

The concept of physical frailty emergence with age due to failure of muscle (sarcopenia, Fried et al., 2001) and cellular energetics (mitochondrial failure; Dirks et al., 2006) has been used to develop a model for physical processes leading to the acquisition of chronic disability. Fried and Walston (1999) proposed a "cycle of frailty" involving the functional de-evolution of interacting "systems" by assessing data on the elderly population studied in the Cardiovascular Health Survey. In that study, Walston et al (2002) evaluated the relation of frailty to diseases present at baseline in older adults, e.g., the prevalence of cardiovascular disease (CVD), congestive heart failure, diabetes, and hypertension. In Figure 1 a schematic of this cycle due to Fried et al. (2001) and Walston (2004) is presented.

Figure 1 shows a complex feedback loop with exogenous inputs that influence an internal environment controlling energy production and expenditure. The directed cycle or "cascade" acknowledges participation of chemoregulators, growth factors, hormones, and cytokines in frailty, which reflects the role of messengers in generating non-local correlations in tissue changes (Cohen et al., 1997; Fried et al., 1998; Huang et al., 2005). To represent this loop in mathematical terms one needs to parametrically describe the essential components of energy production, cell and tissue differentiation, and energy regulation as they relate to an individual's age specific function and total longevity.

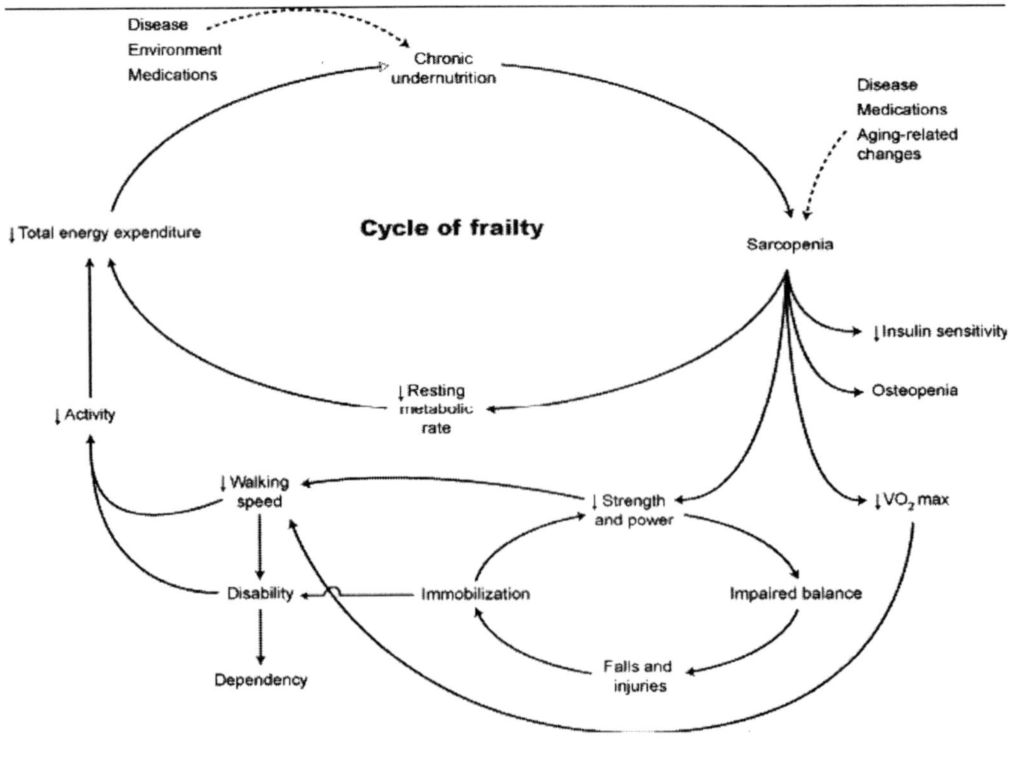

Figure 1. The cycle of frailty. Key components of frailty that appear to underlie its phenotypic manifestations in a negative cycle are (i) chronic undernutrition; (ii) sarcopenia; (iii) declines in strength, power, and exercise tolerance; and (iv) declines in activity and total energy expenditure. Factors that could precipitate or exacerbate this core are indicated with a dashed line. VO_2 max, maximum oxygen consumption.

Clinically, frailty has been defined as physiological vulnerability to morbidity and mortality (Buchner and Wagner, 1992; Fried et al., 1993). Frail individuals are at risk for adverse health events, e.g., falls, fractures, infections, manifestation of disabilities, hospitalization, institutionalization, and death compared to age-matched nonfrail counterparts (Fried et al., 1993; Fried et al., 2001). Although physical frailty is associated with age, disease and disability, those factors don't unambiguously identify persons at high risk (Fried et al., 1998, 2001; Robine and Michel, 2004). Frailty is argued to predict adverse health outcomes independent of age and chronic disability (Fried et al., 2001; Jarrett et al., 1995; Walston et al., 2002).

Thus, to describe the temporal evolution of mechanisms underlying frailty and senescence, and to develop interventions in the frailty cascade, (and to forecast their likely effects), one must have a population model of frailty consistent with frailty processes within individuals so as to be able integrate data, derived from different observational systems across multiple biological levels (e.g., longitudinal studies of general human populations; clinical and epidemiological data; laboratory studies of animal models and experiments on molecular mechanisms). Intrinsic to generating a frailty model is the recognition that frailty connotes a diminished energy production capability and, consequently, because of a lower level of energy resources to respond to environmental stressors increased morbidity, disability, and mortality (e.g., Campbell and Buchner, 1997; Seeman et al., 1997; Simms, 1942; Walston, 2004). It is, however, the frailty cascade involving the multi-dimensional and graded interdependence of the multidimensional interactions of "failing" functional systems that must be described – not the interaction/competing risks of discrete (black box) clinical diagnoses. Disease "categories" only provide a crude basis from which to describe the physiological interaction and competition for internal resources over time of the "true" failure mechanisms (Manton and Stallard, 1988). Thus, a frailty model must describe not only changes in individuals but the dynamic, age dependent parametric coupling of biological processes operating with energy expenditures at different levels of biological complexity in an individual.

Though the model described above in Figure 1 for physical frailty involves primarily muscle tissue, exercise, and interaction with other organ systems there is reason to suspect that similar logic might be adapted to apply to cognitive "frailty" due to dysfunction of a neuron's energetics and the effects of that failure on neuronal energy production, survival and synaptic operations. First, both muscle tissue and the CNS are highly energy intensive consuming tissues in the human body. Indeed, the CNS is by far the most energy consuming tissue in the human body (consuming roughly 70% of all energy produced by the human metabolism) with also the highest rate of free radical generation (Manton et al., 2004; Huang and Manton, 2004).

Second, the CNS is very sensitive to circulatory dysfunction as was described as the underlying physical frailty in the Cardiovascular Health Study. As a consequence, the generation of physical frailty may have indirect adverse effects on CNS frailty and its emergence, e.g., by the operation of cerebrovascular disease. The correlation of physical and cognitive frailty may also be linked to a number of common degenerative processes, e.g., inflammatory cytokines; lipid peroxidation and dysfunction and effects on cell membranes.

Third, the mitotic index of neurons is generally low in adults and the elderly so that loss of neurons due to apoptosis, which is a very energy intense process, may make it more difficult to replace damaged neuronal cells than, say, replacement of myocytes in damaged muscle tissue. Indeed, it is only recently that the operation of stem cells in three areas of the brain has been identified changing the basic paradigm about neuronal replication and repair.

To assess how CNS frailty might be impacted by the cellular failure of energetics we will examine first the components of a conceptual model of energy production in the CNS, i.e., reactive oxygen species (ROS) effects on telomere length, stress induction of telomerase; SIR2 genes and their relation to the effects of caloric restriction on metabolism, and thyroid hormones and their short and long term effects on mitochondrial genesis, structure and operation.

Then we will examine how such mechanisms might be represented mathematically. We will start with the general neural network formulation due to Hobfield using a spin glass representation of the Hamiltonian for the energy expended in the CNS (Stein, 1992) and then generalize the topology of that neuronal field formalism to more general, non-linear topologies. The purpose of these more general models is to enable a more realistic model of neuronal operation and survival than the simple Ising spin glass formulation (neurons represented by specific genes) often used. The major physical components of that more general model, the telomere, the mitochondria, SIR2 and other silencing genes and thyroid hormone regulation of the mitochondria are first described substantatively before we attempt to integrate then mathematically in more general models.

II. Telomeres, Telomerase and Interactions with Mitochondrial Energy Production

One cell feature important to fitness and frailty in both physical and cognitive terms, and which is affected by cellular bioenergetics, is the telomere (Finch and Kirkwood, 2000; Kirkwood, 2002). Telomeres are DNA sequences capping eukaryotic chromosomes. At birth telomeres contain the sequence TTAGGG, repeated for up to 15 kilobases (kb). The enzyme, telomerase, helps maintain telomere length and can be induced by one of several agents (Lingner et al., 1997). Telomeres stabilize chromosomes and bind to proteins preventing them from being treated as double-strand breaks by repair enzymes. Telomere shortening can lead to DNA translocation, fusion, or rearrangement (de Lange, 1992).

Aviv et al (2003) found in vitro shortening of telomeres controlled by: "(a) initial telomere length in the primary progenitor cells; (b) rate of replication; (c) length of the G-rich 3′ single stranded telomere overhangs (SSOs) (*Huffman et al.,* 2002; *Wright et al.,* 1997), which determine how much DNA is lost per division; (d) telomerase (*Bodnar et al.*, 1998; *Morales et al.,* 1999; *Shay et al.,* 2001), (e) patterns of cell division (fraction of self-renewal vs. generation of transient amplifying cells); (f) factors such as oxidative damage shortening telomere (*Serra et al.*, 2003; *von Zglinicki et al.,* 2000)". Telomerase is both up and down regulated by hormonal and other factors (Mergny et al., 2002).

Telomere shortening may be a factor in both cell aging (Slagboom et al., 1994) and low dose IR damage – a process hypothesized to be an excellent model for accelerated physiological aging. Premature senescence in the telomere model is argued to occur at a cell doubling (PD) limit far below the cell- specific theoretical "Hayflick" limit to cell doubling determined from empirical studies (e.g., Martin et al., 1970). To test whether the telomeres' contribution to aging is genetically regulated, Slagboom et al (1994) measured terminal restriction fragments in HaeIII-digested genomic DNA from 123 MZ and DZ twin pairs from 2 to 95 years of age. In Sjöberg et al., (2005) telomeres lost 31bp/year of life. In 115 sets of twins aged 2 to 63 years TRF length was estimated to be 78% hereditable. In Allsopp et al., (1992) the telomere-stress relation was less clear with 15bp lost per year of life in persons aged 0 to 93 years.

Cawthon et al (2003) used quantitative PCR to measure telomere length. Healthy people older than 60 with shorter telomeres showed an 86% higher death rate, and a threefold higher risk of heart disease death and an eight-fold higher risk of infectious disease deaths (primarily pneumonia) than similarly aged people with longer telomeres.

Cherif et al (2003) determined the proportion of telomeres in molecular size regions and not by measuring average length. The latter procedure didn't detect telomere shortening. The proportion of short telomeres increased with age in the kidney, liver, pancreas and lung of male and female rats, but interestingly, not in the brain. Males had shorter telomeres than females in all organs except the brain. Similar findings were reported in mice (Gina et al., 1997) and humans (Melk et al., 2000). This may be due to neurons in the brain generally not expressing a high mitotic index. Gender differences in telomere length in non CNS tissues may help explain female human's longer lifespan (Franceschi et al., 2000; Guralnik et al., 2000).

The change in telomere length, though potentially relevant to a model of CNS frailty, is not sufficient as a model of senescence, bioenergetic dysfunction, mortality and loss of cognitive fitness for several reasons. Telomere length varies within and over tissue types. There are cell mechanisms in many human tissues to lengthen telomeres, e.g., telomerase. Telomerase is an enzyme expressed in specific human tissues (e.g., skin, lymphocytes, intestine). It is inducible in lung tissue by cellular injury from smoking and silica exposure (Mauro and Foster, 2002). This makes the lung a prime target for damage due to inhalation of radionuclides in studies of low dose IR (Manton et al., 2004) and in the chemical and mechanical damage due to inhalation of specific asbestos species (Stallard et al., 2004). Finally, the low mitotic index of neurons may counterbalance the antagonistic effects of the high oxidative stress on telomerase in the CNS.

Stem cells, which constitutively express telomerase, normally operate in many tissues including the hippocampus, dentate gyrus, and substantia nigra in the brain. The capacity for expression may exist in most human tissues with telomerase expressed in 85% to 95% of human neoplasia and, in certain tissues (e.g., lung, heart, and hippocampus), to physical and chemical trauma. Telomerase expression is under complex biochemical controls, e.g., estrogens and androgens may cause expression of telomerase while retinoids and p53 may repress it in cellular functional differentiation programs (Mergny et al., 2002).

Evidence on the relation of telomere length to overall human longevity is mixed. Telomere length and replication count was correlated in vitro but not in vivo (e.g., Cristafalo et al., 1998). Often the correlation of age and telomere length was small (Allsopp et al., 1992). Ben-Porath and Weinberg (2004) suggested telomere length alone does not control senescence but suggests it is also controlled by the structure of the telomere cap. Replication senescence can occur due to stress without telomere shortening. They argue senescence is a general stress response program activated by p53 and Rb proteins and hence is related to mechanisms of carcinogenesis. Others (e.g., Economos, 1982) suggest that longevity in humans is more likely limited by mitochondrial injury than loss of replication capacity due to telomere shortening.

III. SIR2 Genes, "Caloric Restriction", Longevity Proteins and NAD$^+$

To understand how telomere function (and senescence and apoptosis) are affected by oxidative stress due to cellular bioenergetics it is important to understand the interface of the telomere, and energy and ROS production in the mitochondria. One important link is through SIR genes and proteins originally identified in yeast, but some of which are also expressed in a well conserved fashion in humans (Cohen et al., 2004; Lin et al., 2002, 2004; Lin and Guarente, 2003). Since SIR proteins are class III histone deacetylases whose actions are driven by the energy in NAD it was felt they might explain the longevity enhancing capabilities of caloric restriction (CR) (Bitterman et al., 2002). Because NAD$^+$ regulates SIR2, it's effects on mitochondrial function, and its involvement in thyroid regulation of energy production, is important.

Guarente (2000) argued SIR proteins linked chromatin silencing, metabolism and aging. He recognized SIR2 is a NAD-dependent histone deacetylase whose silencing function reduces genome instability. Loss of SIR silencing with aging could allow accumulation of DNA mutations, loss of phenotype, and lead to cellular dedifferention and death. In humans two proteins, hSIRT1 and hSIRT3, are well conserved with their functions well characterized.

Koubova and Guarente (2003) speculated a primary factor controlling longevity in vivo is the activity of cystolic hSIRT1 protein. They suggest a reduction in energy production due to CR is reflected by reduced NAD$^+$ production in mitochondria in the CNS which causes neuroendocrine up regulation of hSIRT1 activity to centrally down regulate insulin, IGF1 and human growth factor production, thus increasing longevity by altering energy production and metabolism. hSIRT1 may also reduce apoptosis.

A related issue is how mitochondria energy production is regulated. In yeast CR shunts metabolic activity to the tricarboxylic acid (TCA) pathway, which enhances, rather than decreases, respiration – contrary to what had been thought about CR and longevity enhancement. In yeast a reduction of ambient oxygen from 2.0% to 0.5% models CR. Reduction in glucose use enhances SIR silencing. Also involved was increased production of HAP4 regulating genes involved in respiration. This increases life span by enhancing electron production facilitating re-oxidation of NADH to NAD to enhance SIR2 expression (i.e., NAD $\rightarrow$ gene expression $\rightarrow$ protein transcription $\rightarrow$ gene silencing and increased genomic stability). The shift in metabolism slows use of glucose since it is more efficient (producing 28 ATP molecules by more complete conversion to CO_2) than fermentation in yeast preserving glucose for conversion to carbohydrate and fatty acid synthesis (Lin et al., 2002).

In mammalian cells raised in serum generated from CR sources the expression of SIRT1 (cystolic protein) was twice as high as in freely fed (AL) mice. Higher levels of insulin or IGF-1 in the serum of AL rats down regulated SIRT1 expression in vitro. It was tested whether SIRT1 down regulated apoptosis induced by Bax. SIRT1 and Ku70 worked together to suppress stress related apoptosis due to Bax protein by sequestering it from the mitochondrial membrane (Gross et al., 2001; Schwer et al., 2002). Other SIRT1 targets include p53 and Fox03 (Cohen et al., 2004).

Liu et al (2002a) showed a direct relation of telomere erosion, chromosome function, apoptosis and mitochondrial dysfunction. Mitochondrial dysfunction produced more ROS accelerating telomere shortening, inhibited telomerase production and increased genomic instability linking three theories of aging (ROS, telomere shortening and macro molecular damage). Also important is evidence that mitochondrial function is a prime determinant of apoptosis (Wang, 2001). One mechanism is the role of anti-oxidant proteins in the BCL-2 family resident in the mitochondrial membrane regulating ion channel formation in response to death signals (Gross et al., 1999). BCL-2 may inhibit transport of pre-apoptotic proteins like Bax into mitochondria. Other proteins resident in the inner membrane space of mitochondria are also involved in death signaling pathways (Wang, 2001).

hSIRt3 is a SIR protein produced in the nucleus but, by the operation of enzymes effecting its transport through mitochondrial membrane, is incorporated in the mitochondrial membrane and matrix in 28 and 44 kda forms (Schwer et al., 2002). Even though there are no histones in mitochondria hSIRt3 may suppress gene transcription relevant to apoptosis (Onyango et al., 2002).

Nautiyal et al (2002) studied the effect of telomeres on survival as mediated by mitochondrial function in yeast. In senescent cells with dysfunctional telomerase and shortened telomeres, oxidative phosphorylation genes were up regulated and mitochondria proliferated. This cell survival strategy uses telomerase deficiency responses (TDR), which included genes controlling processes regulating energy production, stress response, protein folding, cell wall maintenance, carbohydrate and phosphate metabolism. TDR shares some features with DNA repair genes but has a significant component involving mitochondrial function. Up regulation of some TDR genes may be a stress adaptive strategy with telomere dysfunction altering the genetic metabolic program to allow the cell to survive. In cells surviving this crisis, after telomeres were stabilized and perhaps lengthened, a subset of energy production genes remain activated.

In the next three sections we examine how telomere dysfunction may affect three important human pathogenic (cancer, heart disease, Alzheimer's) mechanisms potentially leading to death.

a) Cancer; Failure of Growth Regulation and Functional Differentiation

Analyses of telomerase-deficient mice showed p53 inactivation enhances cell survival with short, dysfunctional telomeres and genomic changes driving carcinogenesis (Chin et al., 1999; Wong et al., 2003). Analyses of staged human colon and pancreatic cancers, show an association of telomere dysfunction and chromosomal instability in early carcinogenesis (Engelhardt et al., 1997a, 1997b; Gisselsson et al., 2001; Takagi et al., 1999; van Heek et al., 2002; Wong and DePinho, 2003; Yoshida et al., 1999). Nakamura et al (2000) found different telomere shortening rates in normal and cancer tissues of 44 and 50 bp/year, respectively.

Telomere length determination in cancers may predict benign-to-malignant progression (Hakin-Smith et al., 2003; Hiyama and Hiyama, 2003, 2002). Wu et al (2003) show short PBL telomeres increased risk for carcinomas of the head and neck, kidney, bladder, and lung. Specifically, 313 patients with these carcinomas compared to an equal number of matched cancer-free control subjects showed telomeres were significantly shorter in all four cancers (odds ratio = 4.5) independent of other risk factors. Telomere lengths were inversely associated with baseline and mutagen-induced genomic instability measured in vitro by comet assays. The molecular nature of this interaction was not determined (Wong and DePinho, 2003).

Without expression of telomerase, incipient cancer cells would either undergo terminal growth arrest (senescence), or die when telomeres become critically short (crisis) (Counter et al., 1992). Fibroblasts undergo senescence in vitro when telomeres reach a critical length (Campisi, 1997). Atrophy and cell loss occurs in testes of sixth generation mTR knockout mice (Rudolph et al., 1999), due to p53- apoptosis (Chin et al., 1999; Marciniak et al., 2000).

The alternative-lengthening-of-telomere (ALT) phenotype may be prognostic for some cancers. Hakin-Smith et al (2003) analysed telomerase activity and telomere lengths in glioblastoma multiformes in 77 patients. 19 (25%) had tumours with ALT. Median survival was 542 days (95% CI 114-970) compared to 247 days (224-270) for cases with normal telomeres (p=0.0003). This difference was found to be independent of age. In patients with non-ALT tumours, telomerase activity did not significantly affect survival (median 287 [199-375] vs 236 [230-242] days, p=0.275).

b) Cardiovascular Disease

Studies of human vascular aging and cardiovascular risks found telomere length in WBC inversely correlated with pulse pressure (Benetos et al., 2001; Jeanclos et al., 2000). Dementia, especially due to cerebrovascular disease, is observed linked with essential hypertension and diabetes mellitus (Butler et al., 1993a, 1993b; Skoog et al., 1996) as well as atherosclerosis and dyslipidemia, and is associated with short telomeres (Aviv, 2002; Von Zglinicki, 2001).

Brouilette et al (2003) investigated if subjects with premature myocardial infarction (MI) had leukocytes with shorter telomeres. Age- and sex-adjusted mean TRF length of 203 cases with premature MI (age <50) was shorter than in 180 controls (difference 299.7±69.3 base pairs, P<0.0001); equivalent to controls who were 11.3 years older – suggesting a considerable acceleration of senescent processes in the persons with premature MI. The differences in mean TRF length could not be explained by other risk factors. Subjects in the lowest quartile for telomere length, had MI risk 2.8- to 3.2-fold (P<0.0001) higher than subjects with longer than average telomeres.

Okuda et al (2000) explored telomere attrition as a function of age and atherosclerosis in human abdominal aorta cells. Telomere length, measured by TRF using Southern analysis, was determined in the intima and media of the distal (infrarenal) vs proximal (suprarenal) aorta. Telomere length was correlated with age and atherosclerotic grade. Age-dependent telomere attrition was higher in both the intima and media of the distal versus proximal abdominal aorta. Telomere length is *negatively* correlated with atherosclerotic grade but, after adjustment for age, the relation was not significant. The high rate of age-dependent telomere attrition in the distal abdominal aorta may reflect enhanced cell turnover due to increased shear wall stress.

Samani et al (2001) compared mean length of TRF in leukocyte DNA of ten patients with coronary artery disease (CAD) and in 20 controls. Adjusting for age and sex, cases had mean TRF lengths 303 bp shorter than controls (p=0.002) equivalent in size to individuals with no CAD who were 8.6 years older. Brouilette et al (2003) and Cawthon et al (2003) found reduced telomere length in leukocytes linked to MI, heart disease and total mortality risk.

Leri et al (2001) reported telomerase activity increased 3 weeks after disease onset and then declined in left ventricle myocytes, but not in ECs, SMCs, and fibroblasts in young dogs with deterioration of cardiac performance and dilated cardiomyopathy. Cardiomyocytes coexpressing proliferation marker Ki67 increased during progression - telomerase activity seemed sufficient to preserve telomere length in acute cardiac failure.

Chimenti et al (2003) reported age-related human cardiomyopathy with increased senescence markers, moderate hypertrophy, and cardiac dilation correlated with apoptosis and telomere shortening despite a 14-fold increase in telomerase-competent myocytes and twice as much telomerase activity with respect to age-matched hearts. Urbanek et al (2003) studied tissue from patients with cardiac hypertrophy, due to aortic stenosis with a mean duration of 3 years. There was a 90- to 120-fold increase in telomerase-positive cells but a 2.7-fold decrease in telomere length, i.e., telomere length declined during age-related heart disease and cardiac hypertrophy despite greatly enhanced telomerase activity. Oh et al (2003) reported age-dependent telomere attrition in patients with end-stage heart failure, but no telomerase response.

Diabetics have increased risk of micro and macrovascular disease (Beckman et al., 2002). Telomere length was shortened in WBCs from patients with insulin-dependent diabetes mellitus (IDDM) compared to age-matched nondiabetics (Jeanclos et al., 1998). Since telomere length did not differ between NIDDM subjects and nondiabetic controls, shortening may only occur in WBCs that affect IDDM (Serrano and Andres, 2004). Obana et al (2003) found CAD patients with hypercholesterolemia and diabetes had shorter PBMC telomeres than controls.

A recent model of atherosclerotic change processes that progenitor cells in the bone marrow produced cells which repaired atherogenic damage to arterial endothelium. When those progenitor cells, in animal studies, lost replicative capacity, atherosclerotic changes were initiated (Kravchenko et al., 2005). Similar processes were found in human genetic syndromes leading to premature atherosclerosis. In normal persons, cell repair capabilities were able to preserve circulatory function in the face of adverse CVD risk factor profiles with CVD disease expression occurring when the cell replication capacity was largely exhausted. This exhaustion occurred at higher rates, due to high risk factor exposure levels (e.g., elevated serum cholesterol).

c) Alzheimer's Disease (AD) and Neurological Disorders

Panossian et al (2003) analyzed telomere lengths in immune cell populations, and showed significant telomere shortening in PBMC from AD cases compared to controls ($P=0.04$). Telomere length of T cells, but not B cells or monocytes, correlated with AD status, measured by Mini Mental Status Exam (MMSE) scores ($P=0.025$). T cell telomere length was inversely correlated with serum levels of TNF-α, with T cells not expressing the CD28 costimulatory molecule, and apoptosis.

Zhang et al (2003) analyzed telomerase activity in 187 AD patients, 53 cases with vascular dementia, and 80 age-matched healthy controls using PCR ELISA. They examined PBMC proliferation in 10 patients with AD and 10 age-matched healthy controls using [3H] thymidine incorporation. Telomerase activity of phytohemagglutinin-activated lymphocytes in AD was elevated compared to healthy controls ($P < 0.01$) and vascular dementia patients ($P < 0.01$). There was a significant correlation between telomerase activity of lymphocytes and dementia severity. The proliferation responses of PBMC to phytohemagglutinin was decreased in AD patients compared with age-matched healthy controls ($P < 0.01$).

Telomere shortening and enhanced apoptosis has also been implicated in the development of Parkinson's disease. The role of various chemical toxins in the risk of Parkinson is suggestive of the effect of oxidative stress on telomeres in the affected tissue as well as the disruption of stem cells producing dopamine producing cells in the substantia nigra. Evidence of mitochondria dysfunction is also found in ALS, progressive super nuclear policy and multi-system atrophy and in Huntingdon's disease (Huang and Manton, 2005).

IV. T3 AND MITOCHONDRIAL GENOMICS AND ENERGETICS

Thyroid hormone is relevant to the telomere-mitochondrial apoptosis nexus, affecting the function and number of mitochondria in cells through several mechanisms (Wrutniak-Cabello et al., 2001) which link cell metabolism and development and differentiation programs. This is briefly outlined in Figure 2.

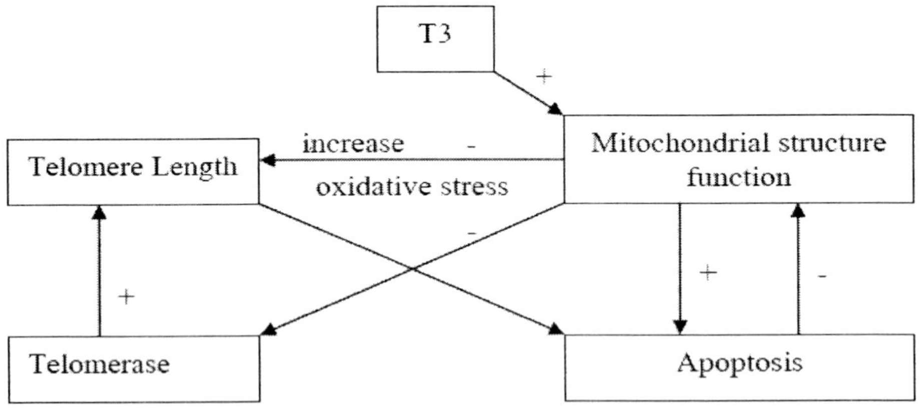

Figure 2. Schematic of the telomere, mitochondria and thyroid feedback for neuronal energy production and apoptosis.

In Figure 2 there are three major components and two ancillary mechanism (apoptosis and telomerase production). One component is the telomere which help regulate apoptosis and cell replication lifespan but which is affected by ROS levels and mitochondrial function and dysfunction. The signs on the arrows connecting various model components suggests the directions (+ increase enhancement of process; – down regulation of process) of the regulation or feedback mechanisms in this model of cognitive/neuronal frailty. The mitochondrial component represents the average state of mitochondria in a neuron in a CNS which is based on the estimated number and functional status of the neuron's mitochondrial population. Thyroid hormone regulates the number and the structure and functional status of the mitochondria in a neuron. CNS frailty reflects the average status of this system/nexus in neurons in the brain both by affecting cell energetics, ROS production and electron leakage and by the role of neuronal loss (death). The intent of the model we will present below is to substitute a model of the average frailty of neurons within the CNS rather than to treat neurons as simple binary operational units in empirical pattern recognition (neural network) models.

The chief regulating factor in the system in Figure 2 is the level of thyroid hormone.

T3 has genomic (changes in gene transcription) and non-genomic effects (e.g., affecting calcium transport (Farach-Carson and Davis, 2003)) on mitochondria. T3 affects cell function through three genomic pathways (Weitzel et al., 2003). The first is a nuclear localized thyroid hormone receptor (TR) which modulates expression of nuclear proteins. Second is stimulation of mitochondrial protein generation through mitochondrial located TR. The third is modulated by intermediate factors which enter the nucleus and regulate secondary T3 target genes. The mitochondrial TR receptor protein P43 increases mitochondrial protein synthesis. Nuclear transcription of mitochondrial proteins is regulated by co-activation proteins which acetylate core histone molecules leading to an open chromatin structure and activation of target genes. If T3 does not bind to a TR then co-repressing proteins, histone deacetylases (like SIR) organize chromatin in a closed form and target genes are deactivated. There is also cross talk between genomic and non-genomic T3 action through activated G protein receptors which rapidly alter metabolism.

T3 receptors in mitochondria affecting short term responses are the 28kDa c-ERB Aa1 proteins in inner membranes. Delayed responses probably result from nuclear expression of genes affecting phospholipids and UCP expression. A 43kDa c-ERB Aa1 protein located in the mitochondrial matrix stimulates the mitochondrial genome. The p43 pathway regulates cell differentiation and is important in organism growth and development (Wrutniak-Cabello et al., 2001). Short term effects of T3 on oxygen consumption have been hypothesized to be due to an effect on a membrane transport protein, ANT, but activity may be instead due to action of T2 on cytochrome-c-oxidase which undergoes conformational changes affecting energy production.

A delayed T3 effect is to increase the area of the inner membrane and change its phospholipid concentrations leading to a 20% increase in proton leakage. Also involved in T3 indirect expression is UCP3 induction affecting mitochondrial membrane function which may be crucial to thermogenesis in warm blooded organisms by uncoupling the rate of respiration from the rate of ATP generation. By controlling the organism's endogenous ambient temperatures UCP3 may affect the activity of many protein-enzyme systems (Wrutniak-Cabello et al., 2001).

T3 increases mitochondrial mRNA levels by 2-8 fold due to increases in mitochondrial transcription factor (mTF). P43, in contrast to the p28 c-ERB-Aa1 receptor, has the DNA binding sector found in the nuclear receptor and efficiently forms sequences of the mitochondrial genome. P-43 activity requires forming a complex with a 45kDa truncated form of PPARγ2 (peroxsaime proliferation activated receptor). Given the high energy level (electron flux) of mitochondria, the effects of IR on the respiratory chain could affect operation of mTF and the generation of mitochondrial proteins in both the nucleus and mitochondria and the operation and function of mitochondria.

P43 governs cell differentiation independent of its effects on energy production and are regulated by coaction with truncated $_{MT}$RXR retinoid receptors in the mitochondrial matrix (Casas et al., 2003). Retinoids thus are cofactors in mitochondrial operation in that they stimulate mitochondrial RNA with p43, help program cell differentiation while down regulating telomerase and telomere length (Pendino et al., 2001). Telomerase activity is generally inhibited by growth and differentiation into a mature state. Effects on maturation may operate independently of the loss of telomerase activity. Telomere length and telomerase expression is under the pro and anti-regulation of steroids, retinoids and Vitamin D as is the expression of mitochondrial genome activity and cell differentiation indicating a complex linkage of multiple steroid signals in controlling energy production and telomere integrity through mitochondrial bioenergetics and gene expression.

This functional complex represents several targets for ROS damage by effects on telomere length and structure, telomerase expression, T3 production and regulation, mutation in mitochondrial genomic activity (which has fewer DNA repair mechanisms and many times the mutation rate of nuclear DNA), hTERT leakage into mitochondria and possibly hSIRt3 (by affecting the NAD/NADH ratio) controlling apoptosis through mitochondrial function.

This complex could be important to understand the pathology in CNS function generated by low dose IR – especially of a Chronic Radiation Syndrome (Akleyev et al., 2000) with symptomatology similar to the chronic fatigue, fibromyalgia and traumatic stress syndromes. The operation of these targets could depend on age related factors (e.g., mitotic index), gender (hormonal status) and tissue burden of metallic ions (e.g., Cu^{++}, Zn^{++}, Fe^{++}) which may be important catalysts in lipid perioxidation in Alzheimer's disease and other neurodegenerative disorders (Manton et al., 2004).

V. Genetic and Epigenetic Modifications of Mitochondrial and Telomere Function

Does awareness of this bioenergetic complex benefit us by suggesting ways to affect those frailty related processes? Or to treat CNS damage due to IR or to chemical toxins.

Standard anti-oxidant therapy (e.g., Vitamin C and E) is not effective in regulation of cellular bioenergetics because of the need to cross the mitochondrial phospholipid membrane and to enter the mitochondrial matrix. Study of the mitochondrial membrane has indicated how therapeutic agents may be transported through those membranes. Smith et al. (2003) and Ross et al. (2005) showed bioactive substances could be attached to the lipophilic triphenylphosphonium cation. These molecules easily penetrate lipid bilayers and, because of the large mitochondrial membrane potential, accumulate in mitochondria.

In a number of studies of aging, whose mechanisms appear to parallel those of low dose IR exposure, combination therapy of the risamer α-lipoic acid and acetyl-L-carntine was successful in reducing both physical and neurological frailty in test animals. The effects, in both cerebral (memory) and physical (muscle strength and endurance) functions, appear linked to an ability to rescue gene expression (RNA) in mitochondria (Liu et al., 2002b). Age related declines in carnitine acetyl transferase (CAT) could be reversed by R-α-lipoic and acetyl-L-carnitine supplementation. The primary mechanism seemed to be preservation of mitochondrial metabolism and energetics by reduction of lipid oxidation in mitochondrial membranes.

Effects of metallic ions (e.g., Zn^{++}, Fe^{++}, Cu^{++}) seemed secondary to production of lipid peroxidation. R-α-lipoic acid, however, has the secondary beneficial effect of chelating metallic ions. Hagen et al (2002) found R-α-lipoic and acetyl-L-carnitine supplements both improved respiratory efficiency (O_2 consumption in hepatic mitochondria) and reduced oxidative stress and liver damage. The increased efficiency of respiration due to acetyl-L-carnitine dictates the need for R-α-lipoic acid because of the need to control increased mitochondrial electron flux.

In addition to the possible intervention in aging/IR related bioenergetic/mitochondrial deficiencies by use of membrane transportable R-α-lipoic and acetyl-L-carnitine, supplementation of L-tryptophan (Bitterman et al., 2002) may improve NAD production, and consequently, efficiency of SIR2 type III histone deacetylase in genomic silencing of nuclear (and possibly mitochondrial) transcription. Study of small peptides (e.g., amino acids like arginine) suggests promise in both control of tissue specific (e.g., NO expression in arterial endothelium) aging and IR related damage (Khavinson et al., 2003; Khavinson and Morozov, 2003; Khavinson et al., 2004).

VI. Energy Landscape Models of CNS Cellular Energetic Models

a) Master Equations and Fokker-Planck Processes

Having described the components of neuronal energy production and, in Figure 2, suggested their logical connection based on those descriptions, the issue becomes one of knowing how to parameterize mathematical models of frailty in the CNS. This obviously requires models of inter-cellular oxidative processes (intra-cellular field effects) and of how the cell is regulated by inter-cellular messengers (extra-cellular field effects). In Manton et al (2004) we used the formulation of a non-linear Fokker-Planck equation specialized to a p-adic random walk, which generated a hierarchical energy field to describe the CNS. In this paper we will try to specialize that general model by taking into account additional specific cellular structures and mechanisms to reflect the average status of the energetic mechanism in neurons, and neuronal death, in a specific individual.

The most general mathematical structure that could be specified for internal cellular protein dynamics requires the specification of the random walk for changes/transitions in the protein system state in cells. System dynamics can be represented by the random walk over the multi-dimensional protein state distribution. Properties of processes describing state changes in individuals, and changes in the distribution of states, define the complex energy landscape over which the random walk is assumed to operate.

At one level this might be described by a reaction-diffusion master equation for a Markov process describing molecular dynamics of J specific chemical/protein species (Isaacson and Peskin, 2005),

$$Q_i(t+dt)=\left(1-\sum_{j\neq i} W_{ji}(t)dt\right)Q_i+\sum_{j\neq i} W_{ij}(t)Q_j dt+o(dt) \tag{1}$$

where

$$Q_i(t) = \text{Prob}\left\{X(t) = i \middle| X(0) = x_0\right\}$$

and

$$W_{ij}(t)dt = \text{Prob}\left\{X(t+dt) = i \middle| X(t) = j\right\}. W_{ij}(t)$$

are state to state transition rates. The coupled ordinary differential equation's (ODE's) where $dt \to 0$ are,

$$\frac{dQ_i}{dt} = \sum_{j:j \neq i} \left(W_{ij}Q_j - W_{ji}Q_i\right) \tag{2}$$

The master equation for stochastic chemical kinetics is,

$$\frac{dP(m)}{dt} = \sum_{k=1}^{K} \left(a^k(m - v_k)P(m - v_k) - a^k(m)P(m)\right) \tag{3}$$

where $a^k(m)$ is the probability per unit time of reaction k for molecular species m. v_k is the change in species for each reaction. These relations are affected by the concentrations of chemical species and stochasticity within each cell (Isaacson and Peskin, 2005). These master equations, however, do not reflect changes in processes due to non-Markovian and non-local field effects. Thus, an alternate mathematical formulation is required to describe CNS frailty.

One very flexible formulation of these processes are the Fokker-Planck equations which describe changes in the distribution of a population of neurons as due to drift (deterministic change), diffusion (stochastic perturbation of individual neurons in the population) and mortality (loss of neurons due to apoptosis). The Fokker-Planck equation can be derived from the general master equations by doing a Kramer-Moyals expansion of the master equation and ignoring terms higher than order three. For complex high dimensional processes, to limit the expression to second order effects one may have to use special forms of the Fokker-Planck equations to approximate the effects of higher order terms by non-linear dynamics and diffusion. This will be discussed in more detail below (Sjöberg et al., 2005).

b) Spin Glass Representation of Neuronal Systems and Neural Network

Biologists often use other types of physical models of energy production to describe frailty in other, but related, contexts (Baake and Gabriel, 2000). A physicist could define energy states for a closed or non-dissipative system using a Hamiltonian matrix formalism. One way to describe the Hamiltonian of a complex biological system is based on Spin Glass Theory, (Fontanari and Stadler, 2002),

$$H(s) = J_{xy}(s_x s_y) \tag{4}$$

where s represents pure states present in the energy landscape and J a scaled state linkage/transition function; H (s) is the energy for state s. States and their relations describe the internal structure of the system and component interactions, e.g., field and frustration effects (high dimensional interactions of states that cause non-linearity in response, and which may increase system complexity; Kolár and Slanina, 2003; Metzler et al., 1999).

These Hamiltonian equations can describe molecular dynamics in a cell, e.g., formation and denaturation of complex polymers, evolution of organization in prebiotic systems, protein dynamics (Stein, 1992). For example, to evaluate the loss of polymer types in a cell one can use the spin glass Hamiltonian where the survival of certain species are frustrated, i.e., aligning some S_i and S_j to be positive makes others negative. The Hamiltonian written to reflect "death" of molecular species is (Rokhsar, 1992),

$$D_N(s) = \sum_{ij} J_{ij} S_i S_j \tag{5}$$

Equation (5) describes the survivability of specific proteins in a cell. To translate protein state transitions, including denaturation, into CNS dysfunction, frailty, and mortality we need to relate individual neuron failure to loss of the capability of maintaining various protein species in a viable state.

These phenotypic functions could be modified to reflect traces over time of what Wright (1931) called fitness, i.e., genetic traits manifest by surviving species (Baake and Gabriel, 2000). In genetic studies of populations, "fitness" applies to success in reproduction – where reproduction has realizations intra-individually at the cellular (neuronal) level which must translate, collectively, to the survival of individuals in a population. This, however, probably has less relevance in the CNS where the population of neurons has a low mitotic index. In our case we, as did Walston and Fried, are dealing with the fitness frailty of a specific organ system, i.e., the CNS. We deal with frailty as the ability of neurons to survive at any age (including after the reproduction ages) as the fitness of neurons in the CNS is lost.

One approach to using the spin glass formulation of Hamiltonians for CNS energy production is due to Hopfield in his evaluation of neuronal networks as models of CNS function. Hopfield used the analogy of neuron function as "on" and "off" switches as reflecting changes in spin as in (4) and (5). This perhaps could model the behavior of cerebral function as a complex bit mapped system with a continuous gradient smoothing the transition from neuron "quiet" to "excited" state. In a Hopfield neural net this function could be logistic in form with the degree of smoothing represented by using a annealing amending approach where the smoothing parameter reflects changing the ambient energy of the system.

In a neuronal system one might consider the Hamiltonian in a three dimensional lattice space with $\sigma_{i\mu}$ represents a spin operation with the values 1 or -1 and with a local field effect, $h_{i\mu}$, producing,

$$H = -\frac{1}{2}\sum_{i}\sum_{\mu \neq \upsilon}\sum_{\upsilon} J_{\mu\upsilon}^{(z)}\sigma_{i\mu}\sigma_{i\upsilon} - \frac{1}{2}\sum_{i \neq j}\sum_{j}\sum_{\mu} J_{ij}^{(xy)}\sigma_{i\mu}\sigma_{j\mu} - \sum_{i}\sum_{\mu}\left(h_{i\mu} + h_{i\mu}^{\text{self}} + h_{i\mu}^{(\sigma)}\right)\sigma_{i\mu}, \tag{6}$$

where we wish to see how external inputs interact with endogenous neuron field structures to generate emergent self organization and increased complexity in the system.

The mean field is given by the local effective field of neurons,

$$H_{i\mu}^{(\sigma)} = \sum_{J \neq i} J_{ij}^{(xy)} m_{i\mu} + \sum_{\upsilon \neq \mu} J_{\mu\upsilon}^{(z)} m_{i\upsilon} + h_{i\mu} + h_{i\mu}^{\text{self}} + h_{i\mu}^{(\sigma)} \tag{7}$$

H refers to what could be called a pseudo Hamilton with the local fields referred as self fields (Inawashiro et al., 1996).

The physiological evidence, however, suggests that the neuron response is strongly non-linear with neurons expressing up to 10^4 inputs with energetics affected both by internal forces (e.g., short and long range (neurochemical)) correlations of activation and inhibition in specific neuronal fields in the CNS as can be generated by the energetic capacity of individual neurons. It is these internal and non-local field effects that we will attempt to model using non-linear mean field formulation of Fokker-Planck equations (Shiino, 2003). In place of the bit mapped spin matrix we will consider a non-linear multi-dimensional transformation of neuronal function to allow more complex topological fields to replace the spin matrix.

c) Topological Changes in the Model

If we define a function, μ_T, as representing the overall frailty of organism *T*, which is a function of the fitness of *K* organ systems, μ_K, we can develop equations both for the increase with age of the frailty of each of *K* organ systems (e.g., the CNS) and the linkage between *K* systems by assuming each operates in an environment defined by *K*-1 other organs. At the lowest level of complexity μ_K is the product of functions describing failure of individual cells (or the failure of specific components of individual cells such as mitochondria or telomeres) due to bioenergetic dysregulation (mitochondrial dysfunction due to IR or other toxic stresses; the effects of ROS in a cascade of failure of other neuronal components, e.g., the telomere and apoptosis initiation) in a specific tissue such as the CNS.

Fitness and frailty is thus multi-dimensional recognizing functional differentiation of tissues with different protein profiles, epigenetic factors, structural differentiation and signaling mechanisms as expressed in Figure 1. One of the characteristic features of the CNS is the lower mitotic index, and longer cell life of neurons – though recent data suggests there are stem cell active areas in the CNS so brain repair capacity is much higher than had been previously hypothesized.

"Genome space", into which the physiological fitness/frailty of an individual can be projected (Kolár and Slanina, 2003), can be described by mutations represented as jumps on a hypercube assuming mutations occur one at a time and to "nearest neighbors" assuming genes are discrete entities. Since fitness evolves in a dynamic phenotypic space determined by interaction of the genome space and internal and external environments, landscape models with multiple time scales and different topologies at different scales are needed (Baake and Gabriel, 2000).

The topology of states described by discrete nuclear mutations is overly simple. A more complete model might be described by a random walk on a hierarchical energy landscape described by the master equation for an ultrametric diffusion process (Avetisov et al., 2002). The master equation is generated by using the Parisi state transition matrix and taking the number of states to the limit to obtain the continuous form of the transition function (Manton et al., 2004). Though continuous that space may be highly irregular or "rugged" depending on the "ambient temperature" (mean particle velocity or energy) and assumptions about how temperatures affects state movements, i.e., the density and rigidity of the particles in the system, (and whether they have internal potential energy) can affect characteristics of movement and diffusion (Chapman and Cowling, 1970). Thus, the master equation would not be well approximated by a Gaussian process such as the standard Fokker-Planck equation (Woodbury and Manton, 1977).

Ultrametric processes (as generated by p-adic random walk) generate a tree like relation of states at different energy levels with movement between states involving energy changes. One use of such analyses, when traits are generated by a clustering of attributes, is to examine the evolution of genes (neurons in our example) with distances between gene (neuron) states reflecting elapse of evolutionary energy/time between emergence of gene clusters (Manton, 1999). That is, one has to conceptually relate the genotypic and phenotypic energy fields as modified by stochasticity and external stressors Generally such dendograms are evaluated topologically without solving differential equations describing the state dynamic processes underlying the dendograms. This inhibits the use of ancillary theoretical and quantitative information in analyses.

In Avetisov et al's (2002) formulation of the ultrametric master equation the ambient energy of the space, which determines it's "ruggedness" (i.e., relative height of energy peaks and valleys), is scaled by an Arrhenius constant based on the Boltzmann distribution which assumes the dynamics of a non-dense gas, i.e., a random walk over a regular lattice. This may be a problem because energy state clusters, in an ultrametric space, are assumed not to overlap (Austin and Chen, 1992). Chapman-Enskog models of dense/mixed gases might be more appropriate in selecting ambient energy parameters controlling an "annealing" process, i.e., smoothing of the energy field topology due to changes in diffusion parameters where interacting particles or structures are not rigid, have internal energy and are of large scale (coarse granularity) for the system. Fontanari and Stadler (2002) found that, for higher energy levels, the trees become unbalanced violating ultrametricity. Alternately one might adopt a random walk on a Bethe lattice to model a "holey" landscape with entire regions inconsistent with "survival" at the molecular level due to thermal protein denaturation (Kolár and Slanina, 2003).

To use a Bethe lattice as the model for a dynamic process requires representing its properties metrically -- most analyses using Bethe lattices (e.g., electron orbitals) are restricted to evaluating topological traits (orbital number). Analogously analyses of metabolomics often use clustering procedures to generate a dendogram of gene clusters reflecting determinants of specific cellular functions without an explicit master equation to rationalize the functional metric relations of gene, clusters or "metagenes" (Dobra et al.,

2004) and energetic networks and may produce anomalous results. For example, two points on a complex protein may be close in Euclidean space but distant in terms of chemical reaction propensity (adapted from Brockmann and Geisel, 2003, Figure 1).

To model such topological conditions the geodesic characteristics of the Bethe lattice (or more generally, of a Husimi "cactus"), may be described by projecting traits on to a hyperbolic space (de Miranda-Neto and Moraes, 1993, 1995). Hyperbolic functions are often used in modeling tertiary protein structures (Zhang et al., 2002). The projective representation of the space is on a Poincaire disk (see b).

d) General Metric Estimation for Systems of Neurons with Complex Structure

The practical question that arises is how to estimate individual positions in such a non-linear state space whose change can then be modeled as a stochastic process. Such a space might be empirically constructed by use of a generalization of the GoM model (Manton et al., 1994). The standard GoM model is described by a bilinear form with convexity constraints on the parameters,

$$\text{Prob}\left(y_{ijl} = 1.0\right) = \sum_{K} g_{ik} \lambda_{kjl} \tag{8}$$

where y_{ijl} are binary measured variables. These might be viewed as neurons with the probability representing the likelihood that they are activated or inactivated. The structural parameters, λ_{kjl}, define K "ideal" or pure state variables (such as the s in spin glass formalism) expressed in terms of the coordinates $\left(\lambda_{kjl}\right)$ on the measures y_{ijl}. The g_{ik} are constrained to a convex space ($0.0 \leq g_{ik} \leq 1.0$) defined by the λ_{kjl} coordinates in the measure space. The definition of the measures depends on biological scale. For protein structures it could be a binary distance matrix between features of the protein's tertiary structure. Likewise the model could be used to evaluate the topology of a neuronal field. The g_{ik} are scores projecting individual states onto the K dimensional convex space identified by the model where the K states defined by the λ_{kjl} in (9) reflect the pure states in the spin model except that they are defined by J attributes of the neuron.

In the generalized model, parameters of the Bethe model would be transformed onto a hyperbolic surface. The generalized hyperbolic GoM equation could then be estimated (Manton et al., 1994),

$$\text{Prob}\left(y_{ijl} = 1.0\right) = \sum_{k,m} \upsilon^{*}_{ik} Q_{km} \upsilon_{im} \tag{9}$$

where the convexity constraints are $\sum_k \upsilon_{ik}^2 = \sum_k g_{ik} = 1.0$ so υ_{ik} may now be viewed as probability amplitudes; Q reflects the matrix of covariances of the probability amplitudes. By appropriate determination of the metric in (10). one can deal with various non-linear transforms –metrics used to describe protein (here neuron) landscapes (e.g., Stec and Kreinovich, 2004) are often projected into hyperbolic space.

The advantage of the generalized GoM representation is that clusters of states (here local neuron fields) need not be non-overlapping (as required in ultrametric processes) – only the extreme, theoretical, or "pure" (possibly unobserved) states defining the boundary of the convex space are assumed not to overlap (i.e., $g_{ik} = 1.0$ or 0.0). By using the parameters, the g_{ik}'s and λ_{kjl}'s (or υ_{ik}'s and Q), in a system of dynamic equations (e.g., the appropriate non-linear Fokker-Planck equation), one can simultaneously define states, and dynamics of states, using the "Heisenberg picture" where state space dimensions are assumed fixed over time (Kovtun et al., 2004; Manton et al., 1994).

Equation (9), can be decomposed into k components using hyperbolic elements to reproduce a high order (up to J) moment structure of the distribution of the elements describing internal neuronal field structure. The number of structures might be defined by the index K. These can more efficiently describe, in terms of a protein landscape model, such topological features as α and β helices, barrels and sheets in protein structures as well as angular orientations. Data of this type can be produced for tertiary protein structures using NMR to reduce crystallographic structures to mathematical coordinates – at this level topology implies function. In other measurement domains this structure may be condensed into functional measures of neuronal fields describing higher level structures (i.e., our telomere, SIR proteins and mitochondrial), losing information, but a loss often necessary for practical analysis. For theoretical vigor the existence of this base protein level must consistently define higher level biological structures and their dynamics.

Alternate estimation methods for dimensional reduction of non-linear spaces using different Minkoski metrics are generically known as multi-dimensional scaling. Curvilinear component analysis is also used to derive a lower dimensional representation of a complex non-linear manifold (Hérault et al., 2002). In genetic and gene expression (RNA dynamics) studies hierarchical clustering into non-overlapping groups would be used to provide an empirical trace of the neuronal energetic processes for which we wish to determine the differential equations –possibly with perhaps different time scales. Both nuclear and mitochondrial genetic analyses have used such procedures to examine processes running both forwards and backwards in evolutionary time (coalescence analysis; Bosch et al., 2001). A representation with non-overlapping groups or clusters is not biologically appropriate if genes share functions with other genes and operate to facilitate other gene's actions. Such phenomena have been labeled degeneracy (different genes performing the same function) and are viewed as an indication of system complexity and may reflect an organism's biologic robustness (Isaacson and Peskin, 2005).

Dobra et al (2004) used a heuristic combination of singular value decomposition and correlations to describe the functional interpenetration of gene groups. In GoM analysis, by reflecting high order interactions in a reduced dimensional convex space, gene interactions and mixtures can be generated more naturally and in a statistically rigorous fashion. By reference back to the formulation of the Hamiltonian of a spin glass model of neural activation this suggests that the states are no longer simply being measured as active or quiet, but represent weighted mixtures of ideal but complex neuron energetic state spaces with a transition matrix to describe the evolution of the continuously mixed space with loss of neurons.

Below we discuss an non-linear Fokker-Planck Ansatz regarding CNS frailty. This will define mechanisms which have to be modeled with data generated at a variety of biological levels or scales (e.g., genetic, gene expression, indices of organ specific enzymatic function like serum cholesterol for HMGCoA hepatic function or of paraoxonase-1 activities, clinical signs and symptoms). Such analyses might help describe the effects of low dose IR on cellular dynamics; or of the chemical effects of specific mutagenic agents on the chemical bond structure of complex proteins.

e) Non-Linear, Mean Field Effect Fokker-Planck Equations of Structured Complex Neuronal Fields

One of the analystic issues is how to translate the spin glass formulation into an equation describing how the probability distribution of neuron energetic states as the distribution changes over time. The classic FPE for Gaussian processes is insufficient to describe how intra-cellular molecular dynamics operating in populations of cells, regulated by populations of genes and genetic elements, filter through layers of biological organization to the distribution of health traits in populations. That description requires models consistent over multiple biological scales. This restricts modeling efforts to models generating "stable" distributions closed under the operation of convolution, e.g., the Levy distribution. Equations, such as the non-linear FPE (Borland, 1998) are needed, that generate Levy type distributions to translate non-local effects over biological scales. Levy distributions imply the existence of Levy flights with state variable velocity and (anomalous) diffusion (Zanette, 1999). Levy distribution frequently emerge in complex biological systems where systems undergo self-organization (leaking) by interaction with the environment.

To describe a population moving over energy states in the neuronal energy landscape, or field, it is useful (as described above) to write a non-linear FPE for changes in the distribution over those states by using a truncated series expansion of the master transition equation (Risken, 1996). Note that the definition of the population distribution, or density function, will vary depending upon the level of biological complexity studied. The population distribution could be the genetic code and its sequence of nucleotides, the population of proteins intra-cellularly undergoing birth (gene expression) or death (thermal denaturation), the population of cells in a tissue with cells undergoing birth, death (e.g., apoptosis) or differentiation, or it could be the survival of individuals in a population. The coupling of these biological levels or organization (i.e., fields with informative structures) requires models more sophisticated than those describing the operation of aggregation and assuming extensitivity because of the presence of a complex set of field effects and interactions at each biological level.

As a consequence of these various factors complex biological systems will not be well described by linear dynamics and Gaussian diffusion. For example, within a cell the gene complement can be better described by a non-linear FPE in that step sizes over nucleotide sequences are constant, reflecting normal diffusion, over coding regions but super diffusive (accelerating velocity of the walk) over non-coding regions (Zanette, 1999). Entropy generating single strand "bubbles" in DNA sequences are more prevalent in areas of weaker adenosine-thymine lines. Transitions across higher energy guanine-cysteine links leads to sub-diffusion (Metzler and Klafter, 2004) as can molecular "crowding" within cells (Weiss et al., 2003, 2004).

These non-linear FPE also suggest the standard Gibbs-Boltzmann definition of entropy does not hold because the assumption of extenstivity (additivity) is violated due to long range field effects and interactions due to a number of physical properties of the system (Borland, 1998). Measures of system dynamic complexity (e.g., Kolmogorov-Sinai entropy) should also be generalized (Latora and Baranger, 1999).

Both "drift" and "diffusion" in FPE could be non-linear with higher order moments expressed in the anomalous different terms as a Levy distribution with complexity characterized by a non-extensive entropy (Abe, 2004). Tsallis (1998) generalized Gibbs-Boltzmann entropy by not assuming extenstivity – local independence of action is destroyed by complex interactions of states. Measures of information and complexity (and its change) can be defined based on Tsallis entropy (Tsallis and Brigatti, 2004) and used to describe chaos and other attributes of system dynamics by generalizing Pesin's identity for Lyapunov coefficients λ_q and of the Kolmogorov-Sinai entropy (Baldovin and Robledo, 2004; Latora and Baranger, 1999). Chaotic analyses of Lyapunov coefficients must also be generalized to evaluate negative eigen-values representing partial self-organizing behavior, or internal control and regulation, in the system. These could be useful diagnostics in the evaluation of the dynamics of neuron fields.

One FPE equation that has the necessary properties to describe the self organization of the local neuron field, and the organization imposed on it by environmental interaction, is a mean field effect FPE, (Bologna et al., 2000) or,

$$\frac{\partial}{\partial t}\left[f(x,t)\right]^{\xi} = \frac{\partial}{\partial x}\left[F(x)\left[f(x,t)+\varepsilon\int xf(x,t)dx\right]^{\xi}\right] + D\frac{\partial^2}{\partial x^2}\left[f(x,t)\right]^{\upsilon} - \mu f \qquad (10)$$

where ε is the average field effect in the "drift" (deterministic) portion of the equation. It reflects coupling of effects between members of a neuronal population. For example, the field effect in (10) could include a "self" field where the local interaction with other spatially contiguous neurons help determine the activity of the index neurons. This would imply neurons do not operate independently. In addition the behavior of a neuron may be a function of its internal state as possibly reflected by the energetic feedback structure as discussed in Figure 2. Non-local interactions could reflect the effects of various amino acid neuro-messengers that affect the threshold of activity of neurons in other, non-spatially contiguous neuron fields in the CNS. The structure, primordial/genetic and acquired, in the field effect, then provides the algorithmic structure of the relation of internal components of neurons and the effects of distant external fields.

Numerical evaluation of (10) may be facilitated by use of Langevin equations (Ito form) (Borland, 1998; Chen et al., 2003), or,

$$\frac{dx}{dt} = K(x,t) + \sqrt{D} f(x,t)^{(\upsilon-1)/2} \cdot \varepsilon(t) \tag{11}$$

The field effect can be generalized to reflect effects operating at different biological scales with multiple field effect terms included in (10) with the coupling of those levels in (11).

A more general non-linear FPE form can be produced by adding a term representing neuronal mortality (Manton and Yashin, 2000) which may be described by an age dependent quadratic function μ of state variables, x, or,

$$\mu(x(t)) = (x^*(t)Qx(t))e^{\theta t} \tag{12}$$

where μ is our measure of frailty, here for CNS function and $e^{\theta t}$ represents the effect of unobserved state variables correlated with age.

State variables can be defined for multiple biological scales and be linked across scales in (12) via coupled non-linear dynamic equations (Kulminski et al., 2004). $e^{\theta t}$ in (12) represents the effect on specific mortality components (neuron specific failure mechanisms) adjusting for the observed state, $x(t)$, of an age variable mean field effects (Manton and Yashin, 2000). These are unobservable effects of aging, e.g., increased rates of protein denaturation in neurons.

One could interpret $\mu(x(t))$ as the frailty of the individual's CNS – or loss of the potential energy production in the CNS necessary to maintain cognitive health (fitness), and draw an analogy between $D_N(s)$ in the spin glass representation and $\mu(x(t))$ in the state variable description by relating the risk of death in terms of energy depletion leading to disruption of cellular molecular dynamics and internal cell structure. Energy depletion could result from defects in metabolism such that creation and maintenance of neurons in specific CNS tissue systems or fields is disrupted. Rosenberg et al (1973) used a thermodynamic argument about human mortality as a function of thermal protein denaturation in an organism in a system without observed state variables. Defects in energy production could be induced externally or internally by ROS generated by kinetic energy from IR or chemical exposures. A critical, analytic issue is how to model changes in scale and protein state topology (Wolynes, 1996) as one translates from molecular to population levels (Kirkwood, 2002).

It is of interest to speculate whether loss of physical energy generation capacity (e.g., decrease in total number of neurons) could be offset by increased neuronal linkage complexity. In this case the mean field effects would assume greater importance in the function of the CNS with age. It would also be of interest to examine how the information in the complexity of linkage exchanges for physical energy.

VII. CONCLUSION

Frailty in aging is, broadly, a loss of energy production capability involving tissue specific mechanisms. Fundamentally, it is failure of mitochondrial bioenergetics to produce appropriate levels of energy with a consequent inability to sustain organ function manifest by protein denaturation and dysregulation of stochastic metabolic processes. This definition can be specialized to the characteristics of individual organ systems such as the CNS.

To describe the change in CNS frailty with age one obviously must evaluate loss of neurons. However, neuronal loss is highest in late childhood as the organizational complexity of the CNS (i.e., the complexity of synaptic connection of neurons; the information content resident in the topological relations of organ fields) increases. Indeed, certain types of functional capacity of the CNS may increase well into the late 70's or 80's years of age if complexity/information in the "algorithm" complexity of the CNS continue to increase due to increased interaction (and accumulation of the effects of interaction) with the external environment assuming that the metabolic support of the other K-1 organ systems provides a facilitative milieu for such continued evolution of CNS function, self organization and complexity.

Such a view of CNS aging and frailty increases our understanding of its basic physiological mechanisms by going beyond chronic disease clinical classifications by describing pathology as disruption of specific parameters of coupled dynamic multi-dimensional physiological processes. Such knowledge is crucial to describe mechanisms to identify modes of intervention in CNS function. For example, knowledge of the biochemistry of the phospholipid membranes of the mitochondria suggests avenues for intervention in pathology of respiration and ROS generation in mitochondria. Specifically α lipoic acid and acetyl-L-carnitine have appropriate ambiphilic properties to induce changes in mitochondrial function. Such characterization will help in the diagnosis, management and treatment of such diffuse, but prevalent, mitochondrial failure syndromes as chronic fatigue syndrome (CFS) – or when associated with low dose IR, chronic radiation syndrome (CRS). It may also have consequences for more focused neuropathological states such as ALS.

What is implied in this altered model of CNS frailty and possible rehabilitation of CNS function is that the information content of the structure of interventions should be high and be consistent with the internal structure of the CNS. This has been elaborated most completely in the time and dose fractionalization of chemotherapy and radiation to maximize therapeutic effect relative to cell cycle, mitotic index gene define systems and the interaction of organ systems in the treatment of cancers. Similarly informed dose time multi-agent scheduling could greatly enhance the efficacy of the treatment of neurodegeneration diseases or the preservation of neuronal fitness – especially at later ages.

Finally, a model of frailty based on well specified cellular mechanisms will improve understanding of CNS senescence, not as a deterministic temporal process, but as a stochastic, complex of evolutionarily preserved stress response mechanisms. Of importance in studying these stress regulating processes are the uses of natural human population experiments where basic CNS processes are interfered with by low dose IR or low level toxic chemical exposure. These are of interest in that the risk of neurological defect increase at low levels of IR dose suggesting interference is synaptic processing – especially the non-local synaptic communication of neuronal fields (Manton et al., 2004).

ACKNOWLEDGEMENTS

The work in this article was supported by grant Cooperative Agreement No.AG07198-15, "Functional and health changes of the elderly" and Multiple Cause grant from the National Institute on aging.

REFERENCES

Abe, S., 2004. Dilation symmetry of the Fokker-Plank equation and anomalous diffusion, *Phys. Rev. E.* 69, 016102.

Adelfalk, C., Lorenz, M., Serra, V., von Zglinicki, T., Hirsch-Kauffmann, M., Schweiger, M., 2001. Accelerated telomere shortening in Fanconi anemia fibroblasts--a longitudinal study. *FEBS Lett.* 506, 22-26.

Akleyev, A., Kostyuchenko, V., Peremyslova, L., Baturin, V., Popova, I.Y., 2000. Radiological impacts of the Techa river contamination. *Health Phys.* 79, 36-47.

Allsopp, R., H. Vaziri, et al. (1992). "Telomere length predicts replicative capacity of human fibroblasts." *Proceedings of the National Academy of Science* 89: 10114-10118.

Avetisov, V., Bikulov, A., Kozyrev, S., Osipov, V., 2002. p-adic models of ultrametric diffusion constrained by hierarchical energy landscapes. *Journal of Physics A: Mathematical and General.* 35, 177-189.

Austin, R., Chen, C., 1992. The spin-glass analogy in protein dynamics, in Stein, D., (Ed.), *Spin Glasses and Biology*, World Scientific Pub Co Inc, Singapore, 6 pp. 179-223.

Aviv, A., Levy, D., Mangel, M., 2003. Growth, telomere dynamics and successful and unsuccessful human aging. *Mech Ageing Dev.* 124, 829-837.

Aviv, A., 2002. Telomeres, sex, reactive oxygen species, and human cardiovascular aging. *J. Mol Med.* 80, 689-695.

Baake, E., Gabriel, W., 2000. Biological evolution through mutation, selection, and drift: An introductory review., in Stauffer, D., (Ed), *Ann. Rev. Comp. Phys.* VII, World Scientific, Singapore, pp. 203-264, arXiv:cond-mat/9907372 v1.

Baldovin, F., Robledo, A., 2004. Nonextensive pesin identity: Exact renormalization group analytical results for the dynamics at the edge of chaos of the logistic map. *Phys Rev E.* 69, 045202(R).

Beckman, J., Creager, M., Libby, P., 2002. Diabetes and atherosclerosis: epidemiology, pathophysiology, and management. *JAMA.* 287, 2570-2581.

Benetos, A., Okuda, K., Lajemi, M., Kimura, M., Thomas, F., Skurnick, J., Labat, C., Bean, K., Aviv, A., 2001. Telomere length as an indicator of biologic aging: the gender effect and relation with pulse pressure and pulse wave velocity. *Hypertension.* 37, 381-385.

Ben-Porath, I., Weinberg, R., 2004. When cells get stressed: an integrative view of cellular senescence. *J. Clin Invest.* 113, 8-13.

Bitterman, K., Anderson, R., Cohen, H., Latorre-Esteves, M., Sinclair, D., 2002. Inhibition of silencing and accelerated aging by nicotinamide, a putative negative regulator of yeast sir2 and human SIRT1. *J. Biol Chem.* 277, 45099-450107.

Bodnar, A., Ouellette, M., Frolkis, M., Holt, S., Chiu, C., Morin, G., Harley, C., Shay, J., Lichtsteiner, S.,Woodring, E., 1998. Extension of Life-Span by Introduction of Telomerase into Normal Human Cells. *Science.* 279, 349-352.

Bologna, M., Tsallis, C., Grigolini, P., 2000. Anomalous diffusion associated with nonlinear fractional derivative Fokker-Planck-like equation: Exact time-dependent solutions. *Phys. Rev. E.* 62, 2213-2218.

Borland, L., 1998. Microscopic dynamics of the nonlinear Fokker-Planck equation: A phenomenological model. The American Physical Society: *Phys. Rev. E.* 57, 6634-6642.

Bosch, E., Calafell, F., Comas, D., Oefner, P., Underhill, P., Bertranpetit, J., 2001. High-Resolution Analysis of Human Y-Chromosome Variation Shows a Sharp Discontinuity and Limited Gene Flow between Northwestern Africa and the Iberian Peninsula. *Am. J. Hum. Genet.* 68, 1019-1029.

Brockmann, D., Geisel, T., 2003. Particle Dispersion on Rapidly Folding Random Heteropolymers. *Phys. Rev Lett.* 91, 048303.

Brouilette, S., Singh, R., Thompson, J., Goodall, A., Samani, N., 2003. White cell telomere length and risk of premature myocardial infarction. *Arterioscler Thromb Vasc Biol.* 23, 842–846.

Buchner, D., Wagner, E., 1992. Preventing frail health. Clin Geriatr Med. 8, 1-17.

Butler, R., Ahronheim, J., Fillit, H., Rapoport, S., Tatemichi, T., 1993a. Vascular dementia: stroke prevention takes on new urgency. *Geriatrics.* 48, 32-42.

Butler, R., Ahronheim, J., Fillit, H., Rapoport, S., Tatemichi, T., 1993b. Vascular dementia: how to make the diagnosis in office practice. *Geriatrics.* 48, 39-47.

Campbell, A., Buchner, D., 1997. Unstable disability in the fluctuations of fragility. *Age Ageing.* 26, 315-318.

Campisi, J., 1997. The biology of replicative senescence. *Eur. J. Cancer.* 33, 703-709.

Casas, F., Daury, L., Grandemange, S., Busson, M., Seyer, P., Hatier, R., Carazo, A., Cabello, G.,Wrutniak-Cabello, C., 2003. Endocrine regulation of mitochondrial activity: involvement of truncated RXRalpha and c-Erb Aalpha1 proteins. *FASEB J.* 17, 426-436.

Cawthon, R., Smith, K., O'brien, E., Sivatchenko, A., Kerber, R., 2003. Association between telomere length in blood and mortality in people aged 60 years or older. *Lancet.* 361, 393-395.

Chapman, S., Cowling, T., 1970. The Mathematical *Theory of Non-Uniform Gases*, in: Cambridge University Press, Cambridge, U.K.

Chen, L., Nash, P., 2003. Sampling transition path with a one point boundary scheme. *Chemphyschem.* 119, 12749.

Cherif, H., Tarry, J.L., Ozanne, S.E., Hales, C.N., 2003. Ageing and telomeres: a study into organ-and gender-specific telomere shortening. *Nucleic Acids Res.* 31 (5), 1576-1583.

Chimenti, C., Kajstura, J., Torella D., Urbanek, K., Heleniak, H., Colussi, C., Di Meglio, F., Nadal-Ginard, B., Frustaci, A., Leri, A., Maseri, A., Anversa, P., 2003. Senescence and death of primitive cells and myocytes lead to premature cardiac aging and heart failure. *Circ Res.* 93, 604–613.

Chin, L., Artandi, S.E., Shen, Q., Tam, A., Lee, S.L., Gottlieb, G.J., Greider CW, DePinho RA. 1999. p53 deficiency rescues the adverse effects of telomere loss and cooperates with telomere dysfunction to accelerate carcinogenesis. *Cell.* 97, 527–538.

Cohen, H.J., Pieper, C.F., Harris, T., Rao, K.M., Currie, M.S., 1997. The association of plasma IL-6 levels with functional disability in community-dwelling elderly. *J. Gerontol A Biol Sci Med Sci.,* 52, M201-M208.

Cohen, H., Miller, C., Bitterman, K., Wall, N., Hekking, B., Kessler B., Howitz KT, Gorospe, M., de Cabo R., Sinclair DA., 2004. Calorie Restriction Promotes Mammalian Cell Survival by Inducing the SIRT1 Deacetylase. *Science* 305, 390-392.

Collins, K., Wong, J.M.Y., 2003. Telomere maintenance and disease. *Lancet.* 362, 983-988.

Counter, C.M. Avilion AA, LeFeuvre CE, Stewart NG, Greider CW, Harley CB, Bacchetti S., 1992. Telomere shortening associated with chromosome instability is arrested in immortal cells which express telomerase activity. *EMBO J.* 11, 1921–1929.

Cristofalo, V., Allen, R., Pingnolo, R., Martin, B., Beck, J., 1998. Relationship between donor age and the replicative lifespan of human cells in culture: *A reevaluation.* Proc Natl Acad Sci U.S.A. 95, 10614-10619.

de Lange, T., 1992. Human telomeres are attached to the nuclear matrix. *EMBO J.* 11, 717-724.

de Miranda-Neto, J., and Moraes, F., 1993. Metric properties of the Bethe lattice and the Husimi cactus. *Journal de Physique I.* 2, 1657-1666.

de Miranda-Neto, J., Moraes, F., 1995. Symmetry properties of the Bethe and Husimi lattices. *Journal de Physique I.* 3, 29-42.

Dirks A, Hofer T, Marzetti E, Pahor M, Leeuwenburgh C. Mitochondrial DNA mutations, energy metabolism and apoptosis in aging muscle. *Ageing Research Reviews* 2006;In Press.

Dobra, A., Wang, O., West, M., 2004. *Graphical model-based gene clustering and metagene expression analysis.* Submitted for publication to Bioinformatics.

Economos, A. (1982). "Rate of aging, Rate of dying, and the Mechanisms of mortality." *Archives of Gerontology and Geriatrics* 1(1): 3-27.

Engelhardt, M., Albanell, J., Drullinsky, P., Han, W., Guillem, J., Scher, H.I., Reuter, V., Moore, M.A., 1997a. Relative contribution of normal and neoplastic cells determines telomerase activity and telomere length in primary cancers of the prostate, colon, and sarcoma. *Clin. Cancer Res.* 3, 1849-1857.

Engelhardt, M., Drullinsky, P., Guillem, J., Moore, M.A., 1997b. Telomerase and telomere length in the development and progression of premalignant lesions to colorectal cancer. *Clin. Cancer Res.* 3, 1931-1941.

Erosheva, E., 2002. *Grade of membership and latent structure models with application to disability survey data.* Pittsburgh: Carnegie Mellon University (Ph.D. Dissertation).

Farach-Carson, M.C., Davis, P.J., 2003. Steroid hormone interactions with target cells: cross talk between membrane and nuclear pathways. *Pharmacol Exp Ther.* 307 (3), 839-845.

Finch, C., and Kirkwood, T., 2000. *Chance, Development, and Aging*: Oxford University Press.

Fontanari, J., and Stadler, P., 2002 Fractal geometry of spin-glass models. *Journal of Physics A: Mathematical and General* 35, 1509-1516.

Franceschi, C., Motta, L., Valensin, S., Rapisarda, R., Franzone, A., Berardelli, M., Motta, M., Monti, D., Bonafe, M., Ferrucci, L., Deiana, L., Pes, G.M., Carru, C., Desole, M.S., Barbi, C., Sartoni, G., Gemelli, C., Lescai, F., Olivieri, F., Marchegiani, F., Cardelli, M., Cavallone, L., Gueresi, P., Cossarizza, A., Troiano, L., Pini, G., Sansoni, P., Passeri, G., Lisa, R., Spazzafumo, L., Amadio, L., Giunta, S., Stecconi, R., Morresi, R., Viticchi, C.,

Mattace, R., De Benedictis, G., Baggio, G., 2000. Do men and women follow different trajectories to reach extreme longevity? Italian Multicenter Study on Centenarians (IMUSCE). *Aging* (Milano). 12, 77–84.

Fried, L.P., Tangen, C.M., Walston, J., Newman, A.B., Hirsch, C., Gottdiener, J., Seeman, T., Tracy, R., Kop, W.J., Burke, G., McBurnie, M.A., Cardiovascular Health Study Collaborative Research Group, 2001. Frailty in older adults: Evidence for a phenotype. J. Gerontol. *A Biol. Sci. Med. Sci.* 56, M146-M156.

Fried, L.P., Kronmal, R.A. Newman A.B., Bild, D.E., Mittelmark, M.B., Polak, J.F., Robbins, J.A., Gardin, J.M., 1998. Risk factors for 5-year mortality in older adults: the Cardiovascular Health Study. *JAMA.* 279, 585-592.

Fried, L.P., Williamson, J.D., Kaspar, J., 1993. The epidemiology of frailty: scope of the problem, in: Perry, H.M. 3d, Morley, J.E., Coe, R.M., (eds.) Aging, Musculoskeletal Disorders: *Concepts, Diagnosis, and Treatment.* New York, Springer Publishing Co Inc. 3-15.

Fried, L., Walston, J. 1999. Frailty and failure to thrive, in: Hazzard, W., (ed.) *Principles of Geriatric Medicine and Gerontology*, New York, N.Y., McGraw Hill, 1387-1402.

Gina, M., Coviello-McLaughlin, G.M., Prowse, K.R. 1997. Telomere length regulation during postnatal development and ageing in Mus spretus. *Nucleic Acids Res.*, 25, 3051–3058.

Gisselsson, D., Jonson, T., Petersen A., Strombeck, B., Dal Cin, P., Hoglund, M., Mitelman, F., Mertens, F., Mandahl, N., 2001. Telomere dysfunction triggers extensive DNA fragmentation and evolution of complex chromosome abnormalities in human malignant tumors. *Proc. Natl. Acad Sci. USA.* 98, 12683–12688.

Gross, A., McDonnell, J.M., Korsmeyer, S.J., 1999. BCL-2 family members and the mitochondria in apoptosis. *Genes Dev.* 13 (15), 1899-1911.

Gross, A., 2001. BCL-2 proteins: regulators of the mitochondrial apoptotic program. *IUBMB Life.* 52, 231-6.

Guarente, L., 2000. Sir2 links chromatin silencing, metabolism, and aging. *Genes Dev* 14 (9), 1021-1026.

Guralnik, J.M., Balfour,J.L., Volpato,S., 2000. The ratio of older women to men: historical perspectives and cross-national comparisons. *Aging* (Milano), 12, 65–76.

Hagen, T.M., Liu, J., Lykkesfeldt, J., Wehr, C.M., Ingersoll, R.T., Vinarsky, V., Bartholomew, J.C., and Ames, B.N., 2002. Feeding acetyl-L-carnitine and lipoic acid to old rats significantly improves metabolic function while decreasing oxidative stress. *Proc.Natl Acad. Sci.* USA. 99 (4), 1870-1875.

Hakin-Smith, V., Jellinek, D.A., Levy, D., Carroll, T., Teo, M,, Timperley, W.R., McKay, M.J., Reddel, R.R., Royds, J.A., 2003. Alternative lengthening of telomeres and survival in patients with glioblastoma multiforme. *Lancet.* 361, 836–838.

Hérault, J., Guérin-Dugué, A., Villemain, P., 2002. Searching for the embedded manifolds in highdimensional data, problems and unsolved questions ESANN'2002 proceedings - *European Symposium on Artificial Neural Networks Bruges* (Belgium), 24-26 April, d-side publi., ISBN 2-930307-02-1, pp. 173-184.

Hiyama, E., Hiyama, K., 2002. Clinical utility of telomerase in cancer. *Labbreu.* 21, 643–649.

Hiyama, E., Hiyama, K. 2003. Telomerase as tumor marker. Cancer Lett. 194, 221–233.

Huang H and Manton KG. The role of oxidative damage in mitochondria during aging. A review. *Frontiers in Bioscience* 9, 1100-1117, 2004.

Huang, H., Patel, D.D., Manton, K.G. 2005. The immune system in aging: roles of cytokines, T cells and NK cells. *Front Biosci.* 10, 192-215.

Huffman, K.E., Levene, S.D., Tesmer, V.M., Shay, J.W. and Wright,W.E., 2002. Telomere shortening is proportional to the size of the C-rich telomeric 3′-overhang. *J. Biol. Chem.* 275, 19719–19722.

Inawashiro, S., Y. Tamori, et al. (1996). "Hamiltonian formalism for self-organization of formal neurons." *J. Phys. A: Math. Gen.* 29: 7389-7399.

Isaacson, S., Peskin, C. 2005. Incorporating diffusion in complex geometries into stochastic chemical kinetics simulations. *http://www.math.nyu.edu/phd_students/isaacsas/* PREPRINT, New York (ed.).

Jarrett, P.G., Rockwood, K., Carver, D., Stolee, P., Cosway, S., 1995. Illness presentation in elderly patients. *Arch. Intern Med.* 155, 1060-1064.

Jeanclos, E., Krolewski, A., Skurnick, J, Kimura, M., Aviv, H., Warram, J.H., Aviv, A., 1998. Shortened telomere length in white blood cells of patients with IDDM. *Diabetes.* 47, 482–486.

Jeanclos, E., Schork, N.J., Kyvik, K.O., Kimura, M., Skurnick, J.H., Aviv, A. 2000. Telomere length inversely correlates with pulse pressure and is highly familial. *Hyper.*36, 195-200.

Khavinson, V.K.h., Lezhava, T.A., Monaselidze, J.R., Jokhadze, T.A., Dvalishvili, N.A., Bablishvili, N.K., Trofimova, S.V. 2003. Peptide Epitalon activates chromatin at the old age. *Neuro Endocrinol Lett.* 24 (5), 329-333.

Khavinson, V.K.h., Morozov, V.G., 2003. Peptides of pineal gland and thymus prolong human life. *Neuro Endocrinol Lett.* 24 (3-4) 233-240.

Khavinson, V.K.h., Bondarev, I.E., Butyugov, A.A., Smirnova, T.D. 2004. Peptide promotes overcoming of the division limit in human somatic cell. *Bull. Exp Biol Med.* 137, 503-506.

Kirkwood, T.B., 2002. Molecular gerontology. *J. Inherit Metab Dis.* 25 (3), 189-196.

Kolár, M., Slanina, F., 2003. Selective advantage of topological disorder in biological evolution. *Eur. Phys. J.* B 31, 379-384.

Koubova, J., Guarente, L., 2003. How does calorie restriction work? *Genes. Dev.* 17 (3), 313-321.

Kovtun, M., Akushevich, I., Manton, K.G., Tolley, H.D., 2004. "Grade of Membership Analysis: One Possible Approach to Foundations." *Invited paper for Focus on Probability Theory*, Nova Science Publishers, NY (to be published in 2005.) Available at e-print archive arXiv.org, ref. number math.PR/0403373.

Kravchenko J, Goldschmidt-Clermont PJ, Powell T, Stallard E, Akushevich I, Cuffe MS, and Manton KG. Endothelial progenitor cell therapy for atherosclerosis: The philosopher's stone for an aging population. *Science of Aging Knowledge Environment* 2005(25), pe18, June 22, 2005.

Kulminski A, Akushevich I, and Manton K. Modeling nonlinear effects in longitudinal survival data: Implications for the physiological dynamics of biological systems. *Frontiers in Biosciences* 9:481-493, 2004.

Latora, V., Baranger, M., 1999. Kolmogorov-Sinai entropy rate versus physical entropy. – *Phys. Rev. Lett.* 82 (3), 520-523.

Leri, A., Barlucchi, L., Limana F., Deptala, A., Darzynkiewicz, Z., Hintze, T.H., Kajstura, J, Nadal-Ginard, B., Anversa, P. 2001. *Telomerase expression and activity are coupled with myocyte proliferation and preservation of telomeric length in the failing heart.* Proc Natl Acad Sci U S A. 98, 8626–8631.

Lin, S., Kaeberlein, M., Andalis, A., Sturtz, L., Defossez, P., Culotta, V, Fink, G.R., Guarente, L. 2002. *Calorie restriction extends Saccharomyces cerevisiae lifespan by increasing respiration.* Nat. 418, 344-348.

Lin, S., and Guarente, L., 2003. Nicotinamide adenine dinucleotide, a metabolic regulator of transcription, longevity and disease. *Curr Opin Cell Biol.* 15 (2), 241-246.

Lin, S., Ford, E., Haigis, M., Liszt, G., Guarente, L., 2004. Calorie restriction extends yeast life span by lowering the level of NADH. *Gene Dev* 18, 12-16.

Lingner J, Cech R, Hughes T, Lundblad V. Three ever shorter telomere (EST) genes are dispensable for in vitro yeast telomerase activity. *Proceedings of the National Academy of Sciences* 1997;94:11190-5.

Liu, L., Trimarchi, J., Smith, P., Keefe, D., 2002. Mitochondrial dysfunction leads to telomere atrrition and genomic instability. *Aging Cell* 1, 40-46.

Liu, J., Head, E., Gharib, A.M., Yuan, W., Ingersoll, R.T., Hagen, T.M., Cotman, C.W., and Ames, B.N., 2002a. Memory loss in old rats is associated with brain mitochondrial decay and RNA/DNA oxidation: Partial reversal by feeding acetyl-L-carnitine and/or R-a -lipoic acid. *Proc. Natl. Acad. Sci. USA.* 99 (4), 2356-2361.

Liu, J, Killilea, D.W., and Ames, B.N., 2002b. Age-associated mitochondrial oxidative decay: Improvement of carnitine acetyltransferase substrate-binding affinity and activity in brain by feeding old rats acetyl-L-carnitine and/or R-a -lipoic acid. *Proc. Natl. Acad. Sci. USA*, 99 (4), 1876-1881.

Manton, K.G., 1999. Dynamic Paradigms for Human Mortality and Aging. J. *Gerontol: Biol Sci.* 54A, B247-B254.

Manton, K.G., Stallard, E., 1988. Chronic Disease Risk Modelling: Measurement and Evaluation of the Risks of Chronic Disease Processe, in: the Griffin Series of the Biomathematics of Diseases, Charles Griffin Limited, London, England.

Manton, K.G., Volovyk, S., Kulminski, A., 2004. ROS effects on neurodegeneration in Alzheimer's disease and related disorders: On environmental stresses of ionizing radiation, in: *Current Alzheimer Research*, Lahiri, D.K., (Ed.) 1 (4).

Manton, K.G., Woodbury, M.A. and Tolley, H.D., 1994. *Statistical Applications Using Fuzzy Sets.* Wiley-Interscience Publication, John Wiley and Sons, New York.

Manton, K.G., Yashin, A.I., 2000. Mechanisms of Aging and Mortality: Searches for New Paradigms. Monographs on Population Aging, 7, Odense University Press, Odense, Denmark.

Marciniak, R.A., Johnson, F.B. and Guarente, L., 2000. Dyskeratosis congenita, telomeres and human ageing. *Trends Genet.* 16 (5)193-195.

Martin G, Spaque C, Epstein C. Replicative life-span of cultivated human cells: Effects of donor's age, tissue and genotype. *Lab Invest* 1970;23:86-92.

Mauro, L.J., Foster, D.N., 2002. Regulators of telomerase activity. A*m. J. Respir Cell Mol. Biol.*, May26 (5), 521-524.

Melk, A., Ramassar,V., Helms, L.M., Moore, R., Rayner, D., Solez, K. and Halloran, P.F., 2000. Telomere shortening in kidneys with age. J. Am. Soc. Nephrol. 11, 444–453.

Mergny, J., Riou, J., Mailliet P., Teulade-Fichou, M., Gilson, E., 2002. Natural and pharmacological regulation of telomerase. *Nucleic Acids Res.* 30 (4), 839-865.

Metzler, R., Klafter, J., Jortner, J., 1999. Hierarchies and logarithmic oscillations in the temporal relaxation patterns of proteins and other complex systems. *Proc. Natl. Acad. Sci.* 96 (20), 11085-11089.

Metzler, R., Klafter, J., 2004. The restaurant at the end of the random walk: recent developments in the description of anomalous transport by fractional dynamics. *J. Phys. A: Math. Gen.* 37, R161-R208.

Morales, C.P., Holt, S.E., Quellette, M., Kaur, K.J., Yan, Y., Wilson, K.S., White, M.A. Wright, W.E. and. Shay, J.W., 1999. Absence of cancer-associated changes in human fibroblasts immortalized with telomerase. *Nat. Genet.* 21, 115–118.

Nakamura, K., Furugori, E., Esaki, Y., Arai, T, Sawabe, M., Okayasu, I., Fujiwara, M., Kammori, M., Mafune, K., Kato, M., Oshimura, M., Sasajima, K., Takubo, K., Correlation of telomere lengths in normal and cancers tissue in the large bowel. *Cancer* 158 (2),179-184.

Nautiyal, S., DeRisi, J.L. and Blackburn, E.H., 2002. The genome-wide expression response to telomerase deletion in Saccharomyces cerevisiae. *Proc. Natl. Acad. Sci.* USA. 99 (14) 9316-9321.

Obana, N., Takagi, S., Kinouchi, Y., Tokita, Y., Sekikawa, A., Takahashi, S., Hiwatashi, N., Oikawa, S., Shimosegawa, T., 2003. Telomere shortening of peripheral blood mononuclear cells in coronary disease patients with metabolic disorders. *Intern Med.* 42, 150–153.

Oh, H., Wang, S.C., Prahash, A., Sano, M., Moravec, C.S., Taffet, G.E., Michael, L.H., Youker, K.A., Entman, M.L., Schneider, M.D., 2003. Telomere attrition and Chk2 activation in human heart failure. *Proc. Natl. Acad. Sci.* U S A. 100, 5378–5383.

Okuda, K., Khan, M.Y., Skurnick, J., Kimura, M., Aviv, H., Aviv, A., 2000. Telomere attrition of the human abdominal aorta: relationships with age and atherosclerosis. *Atherosclerosis.* 152 (2), 391-398.

Onyango, P., Celic, I., McCaffery, J.M., Boeke, J.D., Feinberg, A.P., 2002. SIRT3, a human SIR2 homologue, is an NAD-dependent deacetylase localized to mitochondria. *Proc. Natl. Acad. Sci.* USA. 99 (21), 13653-13658.

Panossian, L.A., Porter, V.R., Valenzuela, H.F., Zhu, X., Reback, E., Masterman, D., Cummings, J.L., Effros, R.B., 2003. Telomere shortening in T cells correlates with Alzheimer's disease status. *Neurobiol. Aging.* 24, 77–84.

Pendino, F., Flexor, M., Delhommeau, F., Buet, D., Lanotte, M., Segal-Bendirdjian, Retinoids, E., 2001. down-regulate telomerase and telomere length in a pathway distinct from leukemia cell differentiation. *Proc. Natl. Acad. Sci.* U S A. 98 (12), 6662-66627.

Risken, H., 1996. The Fokker-Planck Equation: *Methods of Solution and Applications* (Springer Series in Synergetics, V. 18), Springer Verlag; 2nd edition.

Robine, J.M., Michel, J.P., 2004. Looking forward to a general theory on population aging. *J. Gerontol A Biol Sci Med Sci.* 59 (6), M590-1597.

Rokhsar, D., 1992. Self-Organization in Prebiological Systems: A Model for the Origin of Genetic Information, in: Stein, D., Ed), *Spin Glasses and Biology*, Singapore, World Scientific Pub Co Inc; 101-139.

Rosenberg, B., Kemeny, G., Smith, L., Skurnick, I., and Bandurski, M., 1973. The kinetics and thermodynamics of death in multicellular organisms. *Mech. Ageing Dev.* 2, 275-293.

Ross, M., G. Kelso, et al. (2005). Lipophilic triphenylphosphonium cations as tools in mitochondrial bioenergetics and free radical biology. *Biochemistry* 70(2): 222-230.

Rudolph, K.L. Chang, S., Lee, H.W., Blasco, M., Gottlieb, G.J., Greider, C., DePinho, R.A., 1999. Longevity, stress response, and cancer in aging telomerase–deficient mice. *Cell* 96, 701–712.

Samani, N.J., Boultby, R., Butler, R., Thompson, J.R., Goodall, A.H., 2001. Telomere shortening in atherosclerosis. *Labbtru,* 358, 472–473.

Schwer, B., North, B., Frye, R., Ott, M. and Verdin, E., 2002. The human silent information regulator (Sir)2 homologue hSIRT3 is a mitochondrial nicotinamide adenine dinucleotide-dependent deacetylase. *J. Cell Biol.* 158 (4), 647-657.

Seeman, T.E., Singer, B.H., Rowe, J.W., Horwitz, R.I., McEwen, P.S., 1997. Price of adaptation—allostatic load and its health consequences. *Arch. Intern. Med.* 157, 2259-2268.

Serra V., von Zglinicki, T., Lorenz, M. and Saretzki, G., 2003. Extmacellular superoxide dismutase is a major antioxidant in human fibmoblasts and slows telomere shortening. *J. Biol. Chem.* 278, 6824–6830.

Serrano, A.L., Andres, V., 2004. Telomeres and cardiovascular disease: does size matter? *Circ. Res.* 94 (5), 575-584.

Shay, J.W., Zou, Y., Hiyama, E. and Wright, W.E., 2001. Telomerase and cancer. *Hum. Mol. Genet.* 10 7, 677-685.

Shiino, M. (2003). Stability analysis of mean-field-type nonlinear Fokker-Planck equations associated with a generalized entropy and its application to the self-gravitating system. *Phys. Rev. E* 67: 056118-1-056118-16.

Simms, H., 1942. The use of measurable causes of death (hemorrhage) for the evaluation of aging. *J. Gen. Physiol* .26, 169-178.

Sjöberg, P., P. Lötstedt, et al. (2006). "Fokker-Planck approximation of the master equation in molecular biology." *Computing and Visualization in Science.* In press.

Skoog, I, Lernfelt, B., Landahl, S., Palmertz, B., Andreasson, L.A., Nilsson, L., Persson, G., Oden, A., Svanborg, A. 1996. 15-year longitudinal study of blood pressure and dementia. *Lancet* 347, 1141-1145.

Slagboom, P.E., Droog, S., Boomsma, D.I., 1994. Genetic determination of telomere size in humans: a twin study of three age groups. *Am. J. Hum. Genet.* 55, 876-882.

Smith, R. A. J., Porteous, C. M., Gane, A. M., and Murphy, M. P. (2003). Delivery of bioactive molecules to mitochondria in vivo *Proc. Natl. Acad. Sci. USA*, 100, 5407-5412.

Stallard, E., Wolf, R., Weltz, S., 2004. Morbidity Improvement and Its Impact on LTC Insurance Pricing and Valuation. Session #107PD. *In Record of the Society of Actuaries.* 30.

Stec, B., Kreinovich, V., 2004. Geometry of protein structures. I. Why hyperbolic surfaces are a good approximation for beta-sheets.Technical Report UTEP-CS-04. http://www.cs.utep.edu/ vladik/ 2004/abstr04.html- 15. EL Paso, University of Texas.

Stein, D., editor. 1992. *Spin Glasses and Biology. Softcover ed.* Singapore: World Scientific Pub Co Inc.

Takagi, S., Kinouchi, Y., Hiwatashi, N., Chida, M., Nagashima, F., Takahashi, S., Negoro, K., Shimosegawa, T., Toyota, T., 1999. Telomere shortening and the clinicopathologic characteristics of human colorectal carcinomas. *Cancer.* 86, 1431–1436.

Tsallis, C., 1998. Generalized Entropy-based Criterion for Consistency Testing. *Phys. Rev. E.* 58, 1442-1445.

Tsallis, C. and Brigatti, E., 2004. *Nonextensive statistical mechanics*: A brief introduction. Continuum Mechanics and Thermodynamics. 16 (3), 223-235.

Urbanek, K., Quaini, F., Tasca, G., Torella, D., Castaldo, C., Nadal-Ginard, B., Leri, A., Kajstura, J., Quaini, E., Anversa, P., 2003. Intense myocyte formation from cardiac stem cells in human cardiac hypertrophy. *Proc. Natl. Acad. Sci.* U S A. 100, 10440–10445.

van Heek, N.T., Meeker, A.K., Kern, S.E., Yeo, C.J., Lillemoe, K.D., Cameron, J.L., Offerhaus, G. Johan A., Hicks, J.L., Wilentz, R.E., Goggins, M.G., De Marzo, A.M., Hruban, R.H., Maitra, A., 2002. Telomere shortening is nearly universal in pancreatic intraepithelial neoplasia. *Am. J. Pathol.* 161, 1541–1547.

von Zglinicki, T., Serra, V., Lorenz, M., Saretzki, G., Lenzen-Grossimlighaus, R., Gessner, R., Risch, A., and Steinhagen-Thiessen, E., 2000. Short telomeres in patients with vascular dementia: an indicator of low antioxidative capacity and a possible risk factor. *Lab. Invest.* 80, 1739–1747.

von Zglinicki, T., 2001. Telomeres and replicative senescence: Is it only length that counts? *Cancer Lett.* 168, 111–116.

Walston, J., 2004. Frailty--the search for underlying causes. *Sci. Aging Knowledge Environ.* 2004 (4), pe4.

Walston, J., McBurnie, M.A., Newman, A., Tracy, R., Kop, W.J., Hirsch, C.H., Gottdiener, J., Fried, L.P., 2002. Cardiovascular Health Study, Frailty and activation of the inflammation and coagulation systems with and without clinical morbidities: Results from the Cardiovascular Health Study. *Arch. Intern. Med.* 162, 2333-2341.

Wang, X., 2001. The expanding role of mitochondria in apoptosis. *Genes Dev.* 15 (22), 2922-2933. Review.

Weiss, M., Hashimoto, H., Nilsson, T., 2003. Anomalous protein diffusion in living cells as seen by fluorescence correlation spectroscopy. *Biophy J.* 84, 4043-4052.

Weiss, M., Elsner, M., Kartberg, F., Nilsson, T., 2004. Anomalous subdiffusion is a measure for cytoplasmic crowding in living cells. *Biophy J.* 87, 3518-3524.

Weitzel, J.M., Iwen, K.A., Seitz, H.J., 2003. Regulation of mitochondrial biogenesis by thyroid hormone. *Exp. Physiol.* 88 (1), 121-128.

Wolynes, P.G., 1996. Symmetry and the energy landscapes of biomolecules. *Proc. Natl. Acad. Sci.* USA. 93 (25), 14249-14255.

Wong, K.K., DePinho, R.A., 2003. Walking the telomere plank into cancer. *J. Natl Cancer Inst.* 95 (16), 1184-1186.

Wong, K.K., Maser, R.S., Bachoo, R.M., Menon, J., Carrasco, D.R., Gu, Y., Alt, F.W., DePinho, R.A., 2003. Telomere dysfunction and Atm deficiency compromises organ homeostasis and accelerates ageing. *Nature.* 421, 643–648.

Woodbury MA, Manton KG. A random walk model of human mortality and aging. *Theoretical Population Biology* 11:37-48, 1977

Wright, S., 1931. Evolution in Mendelian populations. *Genet* 16, 97-159.

Wright, W.E., Tesmer, V.M., Huffman, K.E., Levene, S.D., and Shay, J.W. 1997. Normal human chromosomes have long C-rich telomeric overhangs at one end. *Genes Dev.* 11 2801–2809.

Wrutniak-Cabello, C., Casas, F., Cabello, G., 2001. Thyroid hormone action in mitochondria. *J. Mol Endocrinol* 26, 67-77.

Wu, X., Amos, C.I., Zhu, Y., Zhao, H., Grossman, B.H., Shay, J.W., Luo, S., Hong, W.K., Spitz, M.R., 2003. Telomere dysfunction: a potential cancer predisposition factor. *J. Natl Cancer Inst.* 95, (16), 1211-1218.

Yoshida, R., Kiyozuka, Y., Ichiyoshi, H., Senzaki, H., Takada, H., Hioki, K, Tsubura, A., 1999. Change in telomerase activity during human colorectal carcinogenesis. *Anticancer Res.* 19, 2167–2172.

Zanette, D.H., 1999. Statistical-thermodynamical foundations of anomalous diffusion. *Braz J. Phys.* 29, 108-124.

Zhang, Y., Kihara, D. and Skolnick, J., 2002. Local energy landscape flattening: Parallel hyperbolic Monte Carlo sampling of protein folding. *Proteins: Structure, Function, and Genetics* 48 (2), 192-201.

Zhang, J., Kong, Q., Zhang, Z., Ge, P., Ba, D., He, W., 2003. Telomere dysfunction of lymphocytes in patients with Alzheimer disease. *Cogn. Behav. Neurol.* 16 (3), 170-176.

In: Leading-Edge Cognitive Disorders Research
Editor: James P. Tsai, pp. 99-130
ISBN: 978-1-60021-843-9

Chapter 4

DEPRESSION AND PREDEMENTIA SYNDROMES: CAUSE OR EFFECT?

Francesco Panza[a,1], ***Alessia D'Introno***[a], ***Anna Maria Colacicco***[a], ***Gaetano Gagliardi***[a], ***Antonio Capurso***[a], ***Vincenzo Solfrizzi***[a], ***Cristiano Capurso***[b], ***Angelo Del Parigi***[c], ***Richard J. Caselli***[d], ***Pier Luigi Scapicchio***[e] ***and Emanuele Scafato***[f]

[a]Department of Geriatrics, Center for Aging Brain, Memory Unit, University of Bari, Bari, Italy

[b]Department of Geriatrics, University of Foggia, Foggia, Italy

[c]National Institutes of Health - National Institute of Diabetes and Digestive and Kidney Diseases, Phoenix (AZ), USA

[d]Department of Neurology, Mayo Clinic, Scottsdale (AZ), USA

[e]Catholic University of the Sacred Heart, Rome, Italy

[f]National Centre for Epidemiology, Surveillance and Health Promotion, Istituto Superiore di Sanità, Rome, Italy

ABSTRACT

With increasing emphasis on early diagnosis of Alzheimer Disease (AD), clinical research has focused on the identification of risk factors that may be modified at a preclinical and early clinical stage of dementing disorders. Prevalence and incidence of different predementia syndromes vary as a result of different diagnostic criteria, as well as different sampling and assessment procedures. Particular interest in Mild Cognitive Impairment (MCI) arises from the fact that MCI is thought to be a prodromal phase and therefore highly predictive of subsequent AD. Furthermore, many of the risk factors for cerebrovascular disease (CVD) and vascular dementia, including serum total cholesterol,

---

[1] Corresponding author: Francesco Panza, M.D., Ph.D.Department of Geriatrics, Center for Aging Brain, Memory Unit, University of Bari,Policlinico, Piazza Giulio Cesare, 11 - 70124 Bari – Italy,Phone:+39-080-5473685; Fax:+39-080-5478860; E-mail:geriat.dot@geriatria.uniba.it

hypertension, atherosclerosis, and apolipoprotein E (APOE) genotype have also been shown to increase the risk of AD. Both vascular factors and APOE ε4 allele have been associated with higher risk of AD. Some recent studies suggested further that CVD or vascular factors increased the risk of conversion of MCI to dementia. Furthermore, depressive symptoms have been associated with cognitive decline and dementia, but the nature of the temporal relationship remains controversial. In fact, studies have ranged from correlating depressive symptoms with subsequent cognitive decline or dementia, cognitive decline or dementia with subsequent depression, to no association between the two. The principal objectives of this chapter were to examine how we might better integrate the varied perspectives on associations among depression, MCI and other predementia syndromes, and cognitive decline and to illuminate the common or distinct mechanisms involved in these associations.

Keywords: mild cognitive impairment, vascular risk factors, Alzheimer's disease, vascular dementia, APOE.

Introduction

Modest decline in memory, particularly encoding, typically accompanies "normal aging". Slowed speed of information processing, and other deficits of prefrontally mediated cognitive operations including working memory, decision-making, planning, and judgment become more prevalent with advancing age, while other intellectual functions such as semantic memory and fluid intelligence appear to remain unaffected (D'Introno et al., 2004).

Subtle cognitive decline can precede the appearance of symptomatic Alzheimer's disease (AD) by many years (Linn et al., 1995), so that current clinical research has focused on the identification of early diagnostic indices of dementia (Panza et al., 2005; Panza et al., 2006). The transitional phase between mild nondisabling cognitive decline and disabling dementia is an ambiguous diagnostic period during which it is unclear whether mild cognitive deficits predict incipient dementia or not. Adding further to this uncertainty are neuropathology-based studies identifying unexpectedly high burdens of vascular (Neuropathology Group of the Medical Research Council Cognitive Function and Ageing Study) and AD (Goldman et al., 2001) types of pathology in clinically nondemented individuals. In fact, in older subjects, particularly over 85 years of age. the prevalence of vascular factors and other medical conditions that impair cognition increases substantially including chronic cardiovascular, respiratory, and metabolic diseases, and severe sensory deficits (Larson, 1993). Not all causes of cognitive decline and dementia are known, but some studies have suggested that these conditions may be prevented (Solfrizzi et al., 1999; Solfrizzi et al., 2003). Previous work has linked cognitive decline to cardiovascular disease, diabetes mellitus, hypertension, and high or low blood pressure (Panza et al., 2004). Various genetic and non genetic factors known to increase the risk of vascular disease, including apolipoprotein E (APOE) and angiotensin I converting enzyme (ACE) genotypes, total cholesterol (TC), lipoprotein(a) (Lp(a)), diabetes mellitus, atrial fibrillation, hypertension, serum APOE levels, and atherosclerosis, have been evaluated as risk factors for AD and vascular dementia (VaD) (Panza et al., 2004).

In the present chapter we will use the term "predementia syndrome" to identify all conditions with age-related deficits in cognitive function reported in the literature, including a mild stage of cognitive impairment based on a normality model and pathological conditions considered predictive or early stages of dementia (Panza et al., 2005; Panza et al., 2006). Such predementia syndromes have been defined for AD and VaD, but have not yet been operationalized for other specific forms of dementia. One of the aims of this chapter therefore is to summarize current definitions of the preclinical or early clinical phase of dementia. Other objectives of this chapter were to examine how we might better integrate the varied perspectives on associations among depression, MCI and other predementia syndromes, and cognitive decline and to illuminate the common or distinct mechanisms involved in these associations. The relevance of the aims of the present chapter were underlined in a very recent article, the proceedings of the 2003 National Institute of Mental Health (NIMH) conference "Perspectives on Depression, Mild Cognitive Impairment, and Cognitive Decline" (Steffens et al., 2006). The principal objectives of the meeting were to examine how we might better integrate the varied perspectives on associations among depression, MCI, and cognitive decline and to illuminate the common or distinct mechanisms involved in these associations. Specifically, research is needed to clarify whether mood symptoms might be included in diagnostic criteria sets (e.g., MCI and mood disorder), act as a modifier (e.g., MCI with depression), be excluded from the MCI diagnosis, or be seen as 1 of 2 distinct but not mutually exclusive diagnoses (e.g., MCI and major or minor depression) (Steffens et al., 2006).

Predementia Syndromes: Transitional Stage Between Normal Aging and Dementia

Although many researchers have suggested and utilized a variety of criteria for defining cognitive impairment and predementia syndromes, they are essentially common with regard to their aim and theoretical framework in that they (i) refer to non demented persons with cognitive deficits measurable in some form or another, and (ii) represent a clinical syndrome that can be utilized to classify persons who do not fulfill a diagnosis of dementia, but who have a high risk of progressing to a dementia disorder (Winblad et al., 2004).

In recent years, numerous rating scales for staging dementia have been developed. The most common rating scales employed in the clinical arena are: Global Deterioration Scale (GDS) (Reisberg et al., 1982), Clinical Dementia Rating Scale (CDR) (Hughes et al., 1982), Cambridge Mental Disorders of the Elderly Examination (CAMDEX) (Roth et al., 1986), and Comprehensive Assessment and Referral Evaluation (CARE) (Gurland et al., 1982). Each of these scales includes a specific preclinical phase of dementia: "mild cognitive decline" in GDS (GDS=3), "questionable dementia" in CDR (CDR=0,5), "minimal dementia" in CAMDEX, "limited cognitive disturbance" in CARE. Moreover, the Consortium for the Establishment of Registries in Alzheimer's Disease (CERAD) introduced the "possible dementia prodrome" (PDP) term for score equal to 0.5 in CDR (Morris et al., 1993). However, several authors make interchangeable use of these different terms, often without supporting psychometric criteria (Andersen et al., 1997; Andersen et al., 1999). The numerous definitions and diagnostic criteria are confusing, and generate variability in prevalence and incidence estimates.

Many different diagnostic criteria and terms have been proposed over the years to describe predementia syndromes in the elderly (Bischkopf et al., 2002) and are summarized in Table 1. "Benign Senescent Forgetfulness" (BSF) proposed by Kral in 1962 (Kral, 1962) denotes a stable nondisabling memory deficit mostly characterized by the inability to recall data and parts of an experience, such as a name, date, or place.To characterize age-related changes in memory more precisely, a NIMH Working Group in 1986 proposed research criteria for AAMI (Crook et al., 1986) (Table 1). However, the criteria of AAMI do not address progression, and so do not clearly discriminate between subjects who will develop dementia and those who will remain cognitively stable. The utility of AAMI has therefore been questioned. In an attempt to address this, Blackford and La Rue further fractionated AAMI, and added an age criterion (Blackford and La Rue, 1989), but still failed to account for educational background; furthermore, there are no epidemiological studies on the predictive value of these subcategories to date.

In 1994 a task force of the International Psychogeriatric Association (IPA) in collaboration with the World Health Organization (WHO) proposed diagnostic criteria for "aging-associated cognitive decline" (AACD) (Levy, 1994) in which patients score at least one standard deviation (SD) below age and education-based standards (e.g. by reference to norms for elderly people) on neuropsychological tests assessing multiple cognitive abilities (memory and learning, attention and concentration, thinking, language, and visuospatial functioning). Thus, the subject groups identified by the AACD criteria are clinically and experimentally less heterogeneous than those identified by the AAMI criteria. In the AACD criteria there is no age restriction: though the cognitive decline is more prevalent in old age, its onset may occur earlier in life.

"Age-related cognitive decline" (ARCD) is defined by the American Psychiatric Association Diagnostic and Statistical Manual (DSM-IV) as "an objectively identified decline in cognitive functioning consequent to the aging process that is within normal limits given the person's age" (American Psychiatric Association, Washington, 1994), but there are no defined diagnostic criteria, and few epidemiological studies using this definition have been conducted (Rediess and Caine, 1996). "Mild cognitive disorder" (MCD) is included in the research criteria for the International Classification of Diseases (ICD-10) (World Health Organization, 1992) (Table 1). Although the definition of MCD is quite different from that of Mild Neurocognitive Disorder reported by DSM-IV (Zaudig, 1992), these two categories share many similarities (Christensen et al., 1995). The diagnosis of MCD is used only when there is an indication of a disease or condition known to cause cerebral dysfunction.

The Canadian Study of Health and Aging (CSHA) introduced the category of "cognitive impairment no dementia" (CIND) to classify all individuals with cognitive impairment that do not meet the criteria of dementia (Ebly et al., 1994; Ebly et al., 1995) (Table 1). This category includes subjects with impairment caused by medical or psychiatric conditions (delirium, chronic alcohol and drug use, psychiatric illness, depression and mental retardation), and offers the advantage of categorizing several broad but specific categories of cognitive impairment that include but are not limited to memory.

"Mild Cognitive Impairment" was first operationally defined in 1991 by the New York University group based on the GDS (Reisberg et al., 1982) and redefined shortly thereafter at the Max Planck Institute in Germany (Zaudig, 1992), based on the DSM-III-R (American Psychiatric Association, 1987) and International Classification of Disease-10 criteria (World Health Organization, 1992).

Table 1. Predementia syndromes: an overview of terms, definitions, and operational clinical criteria

Term/authors	Definition/criteria
"Benign Senescent Forgetfulness" (BSF) [Kral, 1962]	Memory deficit in elderly characterized by the inability to recall on certain occasions relatively unimportant experiences of the past, equally frequent in both sexes, expression of *senium naturale* opposed to *senium ex morbo* in "malignant senescent forgetfulness"
"Age-associated Memory Impairment" (AAMI) [Crook et al., 1986]	Form of benign senescent forgetfulness characterized by the following criteria: *Inclusion Criteria* Age over 50 years; Complaints of memory loss reflected in such everyday problems; Memory test performance at least 1.0 SD below the mean established for young adults on a standardized test of secondary memory (recent memory) with adequate normative data; Adequate intellectual function as determined by a scaled score of at least 9 on the Vocabulary subtest of the WAIS; Absence of dementia as determined by a score of 24 or higher on the MMSE
AAMI (modified) Age-Consistent Memory Impairment (ACMI) Late-Life Forgetfulness (LLF) [Blackford & La Rue, 1989]	*Inclusion Criteria* Age between 50-79 years; Complaints of memory loss reflected in everyday activities, attested by self-administrated and standardized memory questionnaires. Memory test performance are characterized by the following criteria: AAMI, test performance at least 1.0 SD below the mean of younger adults in a well-standardized test; ACMI, test performance 1.0 SD below the age appropriate mean in at least 75% of administrated tests; LLF, test performance 1-2 SDs below the age specific mean in at least 50% of administrated; Verbal and performance IQ scores between 90 and 130 on WAIS or WAIS Revised.
"Ageing-associated Cognitive Decline" [AACD) Levy (1994) [28]	*Inclusion Criteria* No age restriction; A report by the individual or a reliable informant that cognitive function has declined; Onset of decline must be described as gradual and must have been present for at least 6 months; Difficulties in any one of the following areas: memory and learning, attention and concentration, thinking (e.g., problem-solving, abstraction), language (e.g., comprehension, word finding); visuospatial functioning; Abnormality of performance on quantitative cognitive assessments (for example, neuropsychological tests or mental state evaluations) for which age and educational norms are available for relatively healthy individuals. Performance must be at least 1.0 SD below the mean value for the appropriate population.

Table 1. (Continued)

Term/authors	Definition/criteria
"Age-related cognitive decline" (ARCD) [[American Psychiatric Association, 1994]	It represents cognitive changes that are within normal limits given the person's age. There are not operational definitions, but the following criteria should be met to make a diagnosis of ARCD (33): 1. a score < 24 on the MMSE; 2. a score < 80 on the CAMCOG; 3. absence of dementia, organic amnesic syndrome, delirium and other organic syndromes associated with cognitive decline
"Mild Cognitive Decline" (MCD) [World Health Organization, 1992]	Includes a range of conditions in which subjective and objective loss of cognitive functions is not severe enough to fulfill the criteria of dementia, may precede, accompany or follow a wide range of infectious and physical disorders. *Diagnostic criteria* 1. presence of physical disorder; 2. report of cognitive deficit by the patient or reliable informant; 3. abnormality or decline in performance in quantified cognitive assessment; 4. exclusion of dementia, organic amnesic syndrome, delirium and other organic syndromes associated with cognitive decline
"Cognitive Impairment No-Dementia" (CIND) [Ebly et al., 1994]	Classification of individuals over 65 years with cognitive impairment that do not meet the criteria of dementia. *Diagnostic criteria* 1. exclusion of dementia; 2. a score < 24 on the MMSE; 3. a score < 80 on the CAMCOG; 4. clinical evaluation based on direct assessment of the patient, and neuropsychological and depressive symptomatology 5. This category generally includes subjects with impairment caused by medical or psychiatric conditions.
"Mild Cognitive Impairment" (MCI) [Petersen et al., 1999]	*Diagnostic criteria* 1. Report of cognitive deficit by the patient or reliable informant; 2. Absence of dementia as determined by a score >24 on the MMSE; 3. Intact functional status; 4. Objective impairment of memory function assessed by formal neuropsychological testing

Table 1. (Continued)

Term/authors	Definition/criteria
"Mild Cognitive Impairment"(MCI) International Working Group on Mild Cognitive Impairment [Winblad et al., 2004]	*General diagnostic criteria* 1) Not normal, not demented (does not meet criteria (DSM IV, ICD 10) for a dementia syndrome), 2) Cognitive decline -Self and/or informant report and impairment on objective cognitive tasks -Evidence of decline over time on objective cognitive tasks and/or, 3) Preserved basic activities of daily living / minimal impairment in complex instrumental functions,
"Mild Cognitive Impairment (MCI) syndrome" European Consortium on Alzheimer's Disease (EADC) working group on MCI [Portet et al., 2006]	*Different stages of the EADC MCI diagnostic procedure* *First stage* *General Medical Practitioners, Neurologist, Geriatrician* 1) cognitive complaint emanating from the patient and/or his/her family, 2) the subject and/or informant report a decline in cognitive functioning relative to previous abilities during the past year, 3) cognitive disorders evidenced by clinical evaluation: impairment in memory and/or another cognitive domain, 4) cognitive impairment does not have major repercussions on daily life. However, the subject may report difficulties concerning complex day-to-day activities, 5) no dementia *Second stage* *Neurologist, Geriatrician, Memory Clinics* Which MCI syndrome subtype? *Third stage* *Memory Clinics* Which underlying aetiopathogenic sub-type?

WAIS: Wechsler Adult Intelligence Scale
MMSE: Mini-mental State Examination
CAMCOG: Cambridge Mental Disorders of the Elderly Examination COGnitive subscale
DSM-IV: Diagnostic and Statistical Manual of Mental Disorders, fourth edition
ICD-10; International Classification of Diseases 10th revision
Modified from: Panza F, D'Introno A, Colacicco AM, Capurso C, Parigi AD, Capurso SA, Caselli RJ, Pilotto A, Scafato E, Capurso A, Solfrizzi V. Cognitive frailty: Predementia syndrome and vascular risk factors. Neurobiol Aging 2006a;27:933-940.

In 1992 Zaudig, according to the SIDAM neuropsychological test battery, defined MCI as an impaired cognitive status with a score of 34 to 49 on the SIDAM (SISCO) that cannot be accounted for by dementia or any neurological, psychiatric or systemic disease (Zaudig, 1992). At present, the term Mild Cognitive Impairment and its acronym MCI have been frequently used in studies on the preclinical phases of dementia, although with different and inconsistent definitions (Flicker et al., 1991; Petersen et al., 1999). MCI is a clinical label that includes nondemented aged persons with memory impairment and no significant disability (Petersen et al., 2001; Winblad et al., 2004) (Table 1).

There is now ample evidence that MCI is often a pathology-based condition with a high rate of progression to AD in particular (Petersen et al., 1999; Morris et al., 2001), Therefore, MCI seems to be the appropriate stage for therapeutic intervention and predictive factors of the conversion of MCI to dementia are a subject of intense investigation. In contrast, ARCD and AACD are believed to describe normal aging conditions, without progression to dementia. On the other hand, recent studies showed that many people with neuropathological changes of degenerative or vascular origin did not have cognitive impairment (Neuropathology Group of the Medical Research Council Cognitive Function and Ageing Study, 2001), also suggesting that MCI could not have a neuropathological basis. In fact, in a sample of nondemented elderly individuals, pathologically confirmed preclinical AD was not associated with cognitive impairment or decline, even on neuropsychological measures shown to be sensitive to very mild AD (Goldman et al., 2001). These individuals truly are preclinical in that there is no detectable cognitive deficits despite the presence of neuropathological AD, and detectable cognitive decline already may represent "clinical" AD. In fact, a substantial body of evidence supports the suggestion that MCI largely represents very mild AD (Morris et al., 2001).

In 2001 at the "Current Concepts in MCI Conference" a definition of MCI that more broadly encompassed the clinical heterogeneity of MCI patients beyond memory impairment was proposed (similar to the CIND concept) (Petersen et al., 2001b). Three subsets of MCI were proposed: amnestic-MCI (aMCI), multiple domains slightly impaired-MCI (mdMCI), and single non-memory domain-MCI (snMCI). To date, the criteria for these MCI subtypes have been codified and validated by a few epidemiological studies (Busse et al., 2003; Zanetti et al., 2006; Panza et al., 2006c). Patients with MCI may show evidence of vascular disease (MCI with cerebrovascular disease), movement disorders without diagnosed Parkinson disease (MCI with parkinsonism), neuropsychiatric disorders (MCI with neuropsychiatric symptoms) including either mood alterations (MCI with depressive symptoms) or behavioural and psychotic disorders (MCI with behavioural and psychological symptoms) (Petersen et al., 2001b, Luis et al., 2003). In accordance with the clinical categorization of dementia, MCI subtypes according to etiology (MCI-AD, vascular MCI, or MCI-Lewy Body Disease) have been proposed (Luis et al., 2003).

The more recently proposed multiple subtypes of MCI were intended to reflect the heterogeneity of different types of dementia. However, it remains necessary to reach consensus on the nosological definition and diagnostic criteria of predementia syndromes. In this regard, MCI appears to be a better candidate than others, such as AAMI, ARCD, MND, CIND (Hogan et al., 2001), but still lacks standardized diagnostic criteria (Panza et al., 2005). The definition of AACD seems to be one of the best operational constructs (Levy, 1994), and the recent subclassification of MCI seems to be close to the concept of AACD (Petersen et al., 2001b). Currently, aMCI as originally proposed by Petersen et al remains the most widespread and validated "subtype" with high positive predictive value for eventual "conversion" to AD (Panza et al., 2005).

Actually, the recent subclassification of MCI according to its cognitive features (dysexecutive MCI and amnestic MCI (aMCI) or aMCI and non-amnestic MCI (naMCI): single domain aMCI and multiple domain aMCI or single domain naMCI, and multiple domain naMCI), clinical presentation (MCI with parkinsonism or cerebrovascular disease), or likely etiology (MCI-AD, vascular MCI, or MCI-Lewy Body Disease) represents an attempt to control this heterogeneity (Panza et al., 2006d).

This heterogeneity is related to the actual interpretation of the concept and also to the extensive variations in the methodologies used. The different studies nevertheless made it possible to underline the limitations of the current criteria which do not enable homogeneous populations to be defined, both in terms of MCI subtype and in terms of its mode of progression. The diagnostic accuracy of MCI criteria used in drug trials was low to moderate. It is nonetheless essential, above all, to be able to identify patients with a high risk of progression to dementia. A critical review recently took place in Stockholm, then in Montreal in order to define a new consensus on MCI (Winblad et al., 2004; Gauthier et al., 2005). Modification of Petersen's criteria was proposed during the conference in Montreal.

The European Consortium on Alzheimer's Disease (EADC) working group on MCI has very recently proposed a novel diagnostic procedure with different stages (Portet et al., 2006). The EADC working group on MCI presented the elements for review; MCI may henceforth correspond to the following (Table 1): 1) cognitive complaint emanating from the patient and/or his/her family, 2) the subject and/or informant report a decline in cognitive functioning relative to previous abilities during the past year, 3) cognitive disorders evidenced by clinical evaluation: impairment in memory and/or another cognitive domain, 4) cognitive impairment does not have major repercussions on daily life. However, the subject may report difficulties concerning complex day-to-day activities, 5) no dementia.

These criteria underline the importance of the clinical evaluation, which combines neuropsychological evaluation and family interview in order to detect MCI at the earliest possible stage, but above all to identify a decline in cognitive function. The diagnosis is therefore based primarily on the clinical "impression" and no longer focuses on the memory domain. The cognitive complaint itself has an important role, both in quantitative and qualitative terms. Its prognostic value is, moreover, regularly emphasised. Furthermore, cognitive disorders may have repercussions on complex day-to-day activities. Although the concept of slight repercussions is now recognised, the group acknowledges the absence of adequate tools for the evaluation thereof. Questionnaires evaluating function in the course of the past year or a battery of cognitive tests repeated at 6-month intervals, may be necessary in order to evidence this decline.

The new criteria above all make it possible to identify "MCI syndrome", in a manner suited to standard medical practice. The following two points may then be reviewed: 1) which MCI syndrome subtype is involved?; 2) is the underlying aetiopathogenic subtype identifiable? The syndrome subtype may be recognised as early as the initial evaluation. This may involve amnestic MCI, characterised by predominant impairment of the memory domain, or non-amnestic MCI, characterised by slight impairment of multiple cognitive domains ("multiple-domain MCI"), or correspond to predominant impairment of a cognitive domain other than memory ("single-domain MCI"). Certain diagnostic criteria enabling identification of pre-AD (or "prodromal AD") amnestic MCI were recently proposed: 1) criteria for MCI, 2) evidence of objective memory disorders based on a memory test demonstrating the specificity of amnestic syndrome in AD, namely hippocampal amnestic syndrome characterised by a drop in free recall (Dubois and Albert, 2004). It is important to note that none of the tests are obligatory; likewise, the concept of a cut-off has been dismissed. The diagnosis should not be only based on restrictive psychometric definitions, but in combination with clinical judgement. The psychological and behavioural symptoms have to be taken in account too and should not systematically be an "exclusion criteria" for the diagnosis. Subjects may have depressive symptoms related to cognitive impairment or to the underlying process.

The aetiopathogenic approach follows the syndrome stage. A simple classification, corresponding to the subtypes usually encountered during consultations, may be proposed: neurodegenerative disease (pre-AD MCI, Lewy body dementia or, more rarely, frontotemporal dementia and focal atrophy), cognitive disorders corresponding to vascular lesions (vascular pre-dementia MCI, mixed dementia), dysphoric or dysthymic disorders (anxious or depressive syndrome). Certain elements, such as administration of multiple medicinal products, particularly if this includes psychotropic agents or medicinal products with an anticholinergic effect, or multiple disorders, must be particularly taken into consideration in the aetiological process (Ancelin et al., 2006).

Recent evidence on the clinical course of predementia syndrome and particularly MCI, showed that not all MCI patients have memory impairment as the predominant symptom (Petersen et al., 2001b), and not all individuals with MCI progress to AD (Petersen et al., 2001b; Larrieu et al., 2002; Solfrizzi et al., 2004; Tervo et al., 2004). In a recent longitudinal study with a 3.5-year follow-up, the Italian Longitudinal Study on Aging (ILSA), involving a total of 2,963 individuals from age 65 to 84, free-living or institutionalized, we found a prevalence rate of 3.2% for MCI and a progression rate to dementia of 3.8/100 person-years. (Solfrizzi et al., 2004). In this study, MCI patients were selected on the basis of the memory loss, and so probably included many patients with aMCI, with a neuropsychological pattern more similar to AD than VaD. The breakdown in AD, VaD, and other types of dementia of the ILSA was 2.3/, 1.3/, and 0.3/100 person-years, and among those who progressed to dementia, 60% progressed to AD and 33% to VaD (Solfrizzi et al., 2004). This reflects the heterogeneity of MCI (Panza et al., 2005; Panza et al., 2006b). If MCI is essentially incipient AD (Morris et al., 2001), then factors predictive of AD should bear a similar relationship to MCI and both vascular factors and APOE ε4 allele, as a genetic vascular risk factor, have been associated with higher risk of AD (Panza et al., 2004). If MCI is, alternatively, an unstable and heterogeneous category, few factors are likely to be found consistently associated with it. Our recent findings suggested the second hypothesis (Solfrizzi et al., 2004), but, at present, this question cannot be definitively resolved using current data. In fact, previous findings suggest that, in contrast with clinical-based studies (Petersen et al., 1999; Petersen et al., 2001b), where progression is more uniform, in population-based studies the MCI classification is unstable (Ganguli et al., 2004; Solfrizzi et al., 2004). Thus, the apparent homogeneity of MCI and its progression to AD pathology in clinical-based samples may reflect referral patterns and selection criteria, suggesting that MCI is a heterogeneous descriptor and that the outcome at follow-up depends on which population is studied and how MCI is defined (Panza et al., 2005). In fact, persons who have been referred to a memory clinic are likely to be at a different stage of cognitive decline compared with the cognitively impaired individuals from community samples, because they noticed a memory problem and actively sought help for it (Panza et al., 2006b).

Recent evidence from population-based studies (Di Carlo et al., 2000; Kivipelto et al., 2001a; Lopez et al., 2003, Solfrizzi et al., 2004; Tervo et al., 2004) and case series (DeCarli et al., 2001; Frisoni et al., 2002) suggests that cerebrovascular disease (CVD) and vascular risk factors may contribute to the heterogeneity of MCI (Panza et al., 2006a). In fact, vascular risk factors, such as hypertension, smoking, diabetes mellitus, atrial fibrillation, and the APOE ε4 allele are also associated with late-life cognitive decline (Panza et al., 2004), and so may influence the development of MCI and dementia. Because such vascular risk factors may be modifiable, identification and subsequent management of these possible risk factors may help to prevent, and reduce conversion rates of MCI to dementia.

In the ILSA, the multivariable analysis suggested that as in AD only age was a risk factor for incident MCI, while higher levels of education and serum TC appeared to have a protective effect (Solfrizzi et al., 2004). On the contrary, Kivipelto et al. found that midlife elevated TC serum levels (> 6,5 mmol/L) increased the risk for MCI (OR, 1.9), with systolic blood pressure showing a similar trend (Kivipelto et al., 2001a). In addition, De Carli et al. showed that elevated midlife blood pressure increased the risk for MCI (DeCarli et al., 2001). We did not confirm that elevated TC is a risk factor for incident MCI (Solfrizzi et al., 2004). This discrepancy can be explained by the fact that both TC and blood pressure were midlife determinations (with average follow-up of 21 and 25 years) in the De Carli and Kivipelto studies, respectively (DeCarli et al., 2001; Kivipelto et al., 2001a). Furthermore, in a recent study we found lower TC serum levels in AD (Solfrizzi et al., 2002), confirming the data of cross-sectional and prospective studies (Kuusisto et al., 1996; Romas et al., 1999).

Additionally, in a cross-sectional evaluation in the same ILSA sample, age and myocardial infarction were positively associated with ARCD, while age, congestive heart failure, and stroke were associated with CIND (Di Carlo et al., 2000), supporting the role of age and CAD as risk factors for cognitive decline. In the Cardiovascular Health Study (CHS) Cognition Study, the development of MCI was associated with measurements of cognition and depression, racial and constitutional factors, and CVD (Lopez et al., 2003). In some studies the presence of APOE ε4 allele was associated with memory decline in subjects with cognitive impairment (Jonker et al., 1998; Dik et al., 2000; Traykov et al., 2002). In the CSH Cognition Study, classifying patients as having either aMCI or mdMCI, the presence of ε4 allele was associated to the aMCI only (Lopez et al., 2003). Other studies suggested that APOE genotype has only little impact on the degree of cognitive impairment (Small et al., 1998). Finally, a recent Finnish population-based study with a 3-year follow-up showed that higher age, and medicated hypertension are independent risk factors, but high education is a protective factor for MCI, while gender, elevated blood pressure, diabetes mellitus, APOE genotype, or CVD had no significant effect on the incidence of MCI (Tervo et al., 2004). The considerable amount of evidence above referenced may support the hypothesis that vascular risk factors may have an effect on the development of MCI, but further studies are needed to confirm these findings.

A number of studies have examined clinical and imaging predictors associated with increased risk to convert from MCI to dementia (Petersen et al., 2001), and in the ILSA also vascular risk factors were evaluated (Solfrizzi et al., 2004). Stroke was the only vascular risk factor associated with the progression of MCI to dementia (Solfrizzi et al., 2004). In this study, possibly a follow-up period longer than 3.5 years could have revealed that other vascular factors influence the progression of MCI to dementia. In a recent study, the risk of poststroke dementia (PSD) was high (28.5% in a 3-year follow-up, with most patients during the first 6 months after stroke), with about one-third of patients meeting the criteria for AD and two-thirds meeting the criteria for VaD (Henon et al., 2001). CVD is common in the elderly and is known to cause cognitive impairment (Panza et al., 2006e). However, it is far from clear that cerebral infarction predisposes to AD (Schneider et al., 2004), or even increased one year conversion to dementia (Srikanth et al., 2004).

The likelihood of MCI, as conventionally defined (Petersen et al., 2001), may also be increased by clinical and magnetic resonance imaging (MRI) evidence of CVD (DeCarli et al., 2001) and in association with pathological evidence of severe cerebral atherosclerosis (Riley et al., 2002). The incidence of CIND rises in the first year after cerebral infarction (Srikanth et al., 2004). Furthermore, considerable evidence has documented that CVD is strongly associated with dementia in the absence of AD pathology and also may worse or accelerate cognitive decline in subjects with AD (Vermeer et al., 2003). Given this evidence, it seems reasonable to postulate that the presence of CVD would contribute to incident dementia among individuals with MCI particularly due to vascular pathology.

Nonetheless, in a recent case-series study, 52 MCI patients including many with symptomatic CVD were longitudinally evaluated for 3.1 years. Among the clinical and MRI measures, only hippocampal volume was associated with increased risk of progression to dementia. When neuropsychological measures were included in the analysis, memory and executive function were associated with increased risk of progression to dementia, whereas APOE genotype, cerebrovascular risk factors, clinical stroke, presence or absence of lacunes, and extent of white matter hyperintensities did not predict progression (DeCarli et al., 2004). In another study, 29 patients with MCI of the vascular type were compared with 14 with MCI of degenerative etiology based on the criteria of Petersen et al, following patients over 32 months. MCI patients of the vascular type had a neuropsychological profile characterized by poor performance on tests of executive functions and neurological features of parkinsonism without tremor, supporting the hypothesis that these patients have a distinctive clinical picture that can be identified in a clinical setting (Frisoni et al., 2002).

Therefore, whereas considerable epidemiological evidence suggests that cerebrovascular risk factors are associated with various types of dementia, including AD (Kivipelto et al., 2001a; Kivipelto et al., 2001b; Panza et al., 2004), only limited prospective data exist to support the posited impact of CVD on incident dementia (Wolf et al., 2000; Vermeer et al., 2003). In one of these studies (Wolf et al., 2000), white matter lucencies (leukoaraiosis) assessed with computed tomography were associated with increased risk of progression to dementia in a group of 27 MCI patients. Linear measures of medial temporal lobe were also significantly associated with progression. The authors conclude that both cerebrovascular and AD processes likely contribute to dementia progression among cognitively impaired individuals. In a second study, with a larger cohort (1,015 participants) and a 3-year duration of follow-up, a total of 30 individuals converted to dementia (approximately 1%/year) (Vermeer et al., 2003). Prevalent silent lacunar infarction and incident silent lacunar infarctions were both associated with an increased risk to develop dementia or rapid cognitive decline, although this was particularly true for individuals with incident lacunar infarction (DeCarli et al., 2004).

Our findings on the role of stroke in the progression of MCI patients to dementia in the ILSA sample (Solfrizzi et al., 2004), in conjunction with these previous studies (Wolf et al., 2000; Vermeer et al., 2003), suggest that stroke and CVD play a role in the clinical course of predementia syndrome. In contrast with the results of these studies, the study of DeCarli et al. raises questions about the role of CVD in the progression of MCI to dementia (DeCarli et al., 2004). In fact, as reported above, although it is evident that CVD can be associated with cognitive decline (Vermeer et al., 2003; Panza et al., 2004) and is more prevalent among individuals with MCI (DeCarli et al., 2001; Lopez et al., 2003), CVD did not appear to influence progression to dementia when memory impairment was severe (DeCarli et al., 2004), suggesting that only important cerebrovascular brain injury may have an impact on cognitive function.

Several reports of neuropsychological testing among individuals with MCI suggest that the severity of memory impairment strongly predicts progression to dementia (Petersen et al., 1999; Petersen et al., 2001), and associated deficits in language or impairments in other cognitive domains may contribute to a more rapid progression (Bozoki et al., 2001). In addition to a neuropsychological assessment, as reported above, different approaches have been undertaken to predict the outcome of MCI, such as assessment of plasma β-amyloid, structural and functional neuroimaging, and APOE genotyping. In particular, several gene polymorphisms associated with vascular disease have been found to increase susceptibility to sporadic AD (Panza et al., 2004). A number of studies have looked at the impact of APOE genotype on the risk of progression of MCI to dementia. In a study carried-out in Rochester, the APOE ε4 genotype strongly predicted progression of memory-impaired persons to AD (Petersen et al., 1995). Furthermore, Petersen et al. reported that APOE ε4 allele status appears to be a strong predictor of subsequent development of dementia in patients with MCI (Petersen et al., 1996). In contrast, three very recent studies failed to find evidence of an association of the presence of the APOE e4 allele with progression to dementia in MCI patients or with incident MCI (DeCarli et al., 2001; Ganguli et al., 2004; Tervo et al., 2004). In fact, in a Finnish population-based study elevated blood pressure, diabetes mellitus, APOE genotype, or CVD had no significant impact on the conversion to MCI (Tervo et al., 2004), confirming the controversial findings on this vascular genetic risk factor in MCI. In the MoVIES study, progression from MCI to AD was associated only with age (Ganguli et al., 2004); lack of power is a possible explanation, given the small numbers of persons who met criteria for MCI in these studies. These findings were confirmed by the case-series study of DeCarli and colleagues in which APOE genotype, clinical stroke, and other cerebrovascular risk factors hyperintensities did not predict progression (DeCarli et al., 2001). In our recent study, 209 older subjects (65 patients with AD, 45 patients with MCI (25 aMCI and 20 multiple domain MCI), and 99 without cognitive impairment (NoCI)). In MCI group (aMCI + multiple domain MCI), we found a frequency of APOE ε4 allele similar to that from other nondemented Caucasian populations (Blair et al., 2005). As expected, we found a significant association between the APOE ε4 allele and AD. Moreover, prevalence of ε4-carriers in our AD group was not significantly different from that observed in the aMCI subset (Orsitto et al., 2006). Conversely, multiple domain MCI patients had a significantly lower frequency of ε4-carriers than AD and aMCI groups, confirming previous reports (Manly et al., 2005). The prevalence of APOE ε4 similar in AD and aMCI, but very different from that of multiple domain MCI subset, suggests that a large percentage of the ε4-carriers with aMCI might be predisposed to develop AD (Morris et al., 2001). Further studies on larger samples are needed to confirm the association of APOE alleles with different MCI subsets.

PREVALENCE AND INCIDENCE OF DEPRESSION IN PREDEMENTIA SYNDROMES

Late-life depression refers to depressive syndromes defined in the DSM-IV (American Psychiatric Association, 1994) and in the ICD-10 (World Health Organization, 1992) that arise in adults older than age 65 years. In old age, depressive syndromes often affect people with chronic medical illnesses, cognitive impairment, or disability (Alexopoulos et al., 2002; Alexopoulos, 2005). Beyond personal suffering and family disruption, depression worsens the outcomes of many medical disorders and promotes disability (Blazer, 2003; Charney et al., 2003). Although progress has been made in characterising the presentation of latelife depression and in improving its treatment, it continues to have detrimental consequences (Charney et al., 2003). Given the complexity of this topic, clarity about the term depression is important. For example, not all clinical researchers are in agreement about the term depression when applied to older patients with a mood disturbance. There is likely to be agreement when one takes a syndromal approach to depression, calling on the DSM-IV (American Psychiatric Association, 1994), to identify symptom clusters such as major depression. In major depression, state-of-the-art research assessment relies on the use of structured clinical interviewing as exemplified by the Structured Clinical Interview for DSM-IV (First et al., 1997), to guide data acquisition from many sources about past and current psychiatric symptoms and about past and current Axis I diagnoses. However, other subtypes of depression, including subsyndromal depression in which symptoms are present intermittently (Lyness et al., 1999) and nondysphoric depression in which feelings of sadness are denied (Gallo et al., 1997), may be as important in older adults as major depression because of their association with functional disability and cognitive impairment. In this chapter, depression will refer to clinically significant depressive symptoms and subsumes major depression, dysthymia, and subsyndromal and other subtypes of depression (Steffens et al., 2006). Some elderly individuals develop dementia during episodes of depression that subsides after remission of depression (pseudodementia). Most of these patients have late-onset major depression. Furthermore, a large proportion of those with reversible dementia are left with some form of cognitive impairment after remission of depression, and about 40% develop irreversible dementia within 3 years of follow up (Alexopoulos et al., 1993). Thus, reversible dementia is often an early manifestation of a more permanent disorder and constitutes an indication for diagnostic workup aimed at the identification of treatable dementia.

Late-life depressive syndromes often arise in the context of medical and neurological disorders (Alexopoulos et al., 2002; Alexopoulos, 2005). Symptoms or syndromes of depression are often present in individuals with dementia. The point prevalence of major depression is about 17% in patients with AD (Wragg and Jestem 1989) and is even higher in those with subcortical dementias (Sobin and Sacheim HA, 1997). The US NIMH has developed provisional criteria for the diagnosis of depression in individuals with AD (Olin et al., 2002) to identify the problem and to promote research into the disorder (Table 2). Furthermore, as above-cited, the 2003 NIMH conference "Perspectives on Depression, Mild Cognitive Impairment, and Cognitive Decline" examined the associations among predementia syndromes and depression (Steffens et al., 2006).

Depressive symptoms have been associated with cognitive decline and dementia, but the nature of the temporal relationship remains controversial (Devanand et al., 1996; Bassuk et al., 1998; Yaffe et al., 1999; Geerlings et al., 2000; Paterniti et al., 2002; Wilson et al., 2002; Fuhrer et al., 2003; Green et al., 2003; Wilson et al., 2004; Dal Forno et al., 2005; Gatz et al., 2005; Sachs-Ericsson et al., 2005; Barnes et al., 2006; Geda et al., 2006; Dufouil et al., 1996; Palsson et al., 1999; Ganguli et al., 2006; Chen et al., 1999; Vinkers et al., 2004; Holtzer et al., 2005). In fact, studies have ranged from correlating depressive symptoms with subsequent cognitive decline or dementia (Devanand et al., 1996; Bassuk et al., 1998; Yaffe et al., 1999; Geerlings et al., 2000; Paterniti et al., 2002; Wilson et al., 2002; Fuhrer et al., 2003; Green et al., 2003; Wilson et al., 2004; Dal Forno et al., 2005; Gatz et al., 2005; Sachs-Ericsson et al., 2005; Barnes et al., 2006; Geda et al., 2006), cognitive decline or dementia with subsequent depression (Chen et al., 1999; Vinkers et al., 2004; Ganguli et al., 2006), to no association between the two (Dufouil et al., 1996; Palsson et al., 1999). Some studies found that depression predicted cognitive decline (Devanand et al., 1996; Bassuk et al., 1998; Yaffe et al., 1999;

Table 2. Provisional diagnostic criteria for depression in patients with Alzheimer's disease

Clinically significant depressive symptoms
Three or more depressive symptoms during the same 2-week period, representing a change from previous functioning
At least one of the symptoms must be either depressed mood or decreased positive affect or pleasure. Other depressive symptoms are: • clinically significant depressed mood—eg, depressed, sad, hopeless, discouraged, tearful; • decreased positive affect or pleasure in response to social contacts and usual activities; • social isolation or withdrawal; • disruption in appetite; • disruption in sleep; • psychomotor changes—eg, agitation or retardation; • irritability; • fatigue or loss of energy; • feelings of worthlessness, hopelessness, or excessive or inappropriate guilt; • recurrent thoughts of death, suicidal ideation, plan or attempt Symptoms should not be a result of dementia symptoms—eg, loss of weight due to difficulties with food intake
Depression should not be part of idiopathic depression, other mental disorders, a medical condition, or medication use

Modified from: Olin JT, Schneider LS, Katz IR, Meyers BS, Alexopoulos GS, Breitner JC, Bruce ML, Caine ED, Cummings JL, Devanand DP, Krishnan KR, Lyketsos CG, Lyness JM, Rabins PV, Reynolds CF 3rd, Rovner BW, Steffens DC, Tariot PN, Lebowitz BD. Provisional diagnostic criteria for depression of Alzheimer's disease. Am J Geriatr Psychiatry 2002; 10: 125–28.

Geerlings et al., 2000; Paterniti et al., 2002; Wilson et al., 2002; Fuhrer et al., 2003; Green et al., 2003; Wilson et al., 2004; Dal Forno et al., 2005; Gatz et al., 2005; Sachs-Ericsson et al., 2005; Barnes et al., 2006; Geda et al., 2006), but others did not confirm these findings (Dufouil et al., 1996; Palsson et al., 1999; Ganguli et al., 2006; Chen et al., 1999; Vinkers et al., 2004). Only two population-based studies have investigated the temporal relationship between depressive symptoms and cognitive impairment (Chen et al., 1999; Vinkers et al., 2004). In fact, very recently, depressive symptoms at baseline were not related to an accelerated cognitive decline during follow up in elderly people (Vinkers et al., 2004), confirming findings showing that depression is an early manifestation rather than a risk factor for dementia and AD (Chen et al., 1999). On the other hand, the Predictors Study, a multicenter cohort study with follow-up of up to 14 years, suggested that decline in functional activity but not in cognition precedes the first episode of depressive symptoms in patients with probable AD (Holtzer et al., 2005).

Recently, in the ILSA, in a a population based study with a sample of 5,632 65-84 year old subjects, we found that the diagnosis of MCI was associated with a high prevalence and incidence of depressive symptoms after a follow-up of 3.5 years, with a higher prevalence of mild depressive symptoms and incidence of severe depressive symptoms. We found a prevalence rate of 63.3% of depressive symptoms among MCI: 49.3% had mild and 14.0% had severe depressive symptoms (Panza et al., 2004). Many recent population-based (Lyketsos et al., 2002; Chan et al., 2003; Forsell et al., 2003) or case-control studies (Copeland et al., 2003; Hwang et al., 2004; Feldman et al., 2004; Geda et al., 2004) determined the prevalence of depressive and other neuropsychiatric symptoms among patients with preclinical AD or MCI. Findings have been inconsistent mainly because of different assessment procedures. Although some MCI studies reported a low prevalence of depressive symptoms (Petersen et al., 1999; Geda et al., 2004), the investigators of the population-based CHS report a cumulative prevalence of 26% for depression among individuals with MCI (of the amnestic or the multidomain subtypes) (Lyketsos et al., 2002). The CHS Cognition Study utilized the Neuropsychiatric Inventory (NPI) (Cummings et al., 1994), suggesting an association between depression and MCI (Lyketsos et al., 2002). Accepting some differences in methodology, our prevalence rates of depressive symptoms assessed with the GDS among MCI patients was more than twice that found in the CHS Cognition Study. Furthermore, in the CHS Cognition Study, the development of MCI was associated cross-sectionally with racial and constitutional factors, cerebrovascular disease, and measurements of cognition and depression (Lopez et al., 2003). In another study, those classified as MCI had an even lower prevalence of depressive symptoms: only 15.7% as a NPI symptom in the past month (Chan et al., 2003). In the Kungsholmen Project, a Swedish population-based study, the reported prevalence of depression in MCI was 10% (according to the DSM-III-R criteria): 20% reported loss of initiative, 9% loss of interest, 9% suicidal thoughts, 4% depressive thoughts, and 11% reported sadness,8 as rated using the Comprehensive Psychopathological Rating Scale (Asberg et al., 1979).

In a recent case-control study, nondemented subjects who progressed to AD over a 3-year period had more depressive symptoms and symptoms of personality changes (such as agitation and passivity) at baseline than those who did not progress to AD (Copeland et al., 2003). Furthermore, Hwang and colleagues found that the most significant differences between MCI and controls were mood symptoms, including dysphoria, anxiety, and irritability (Hwang et al., 2004). Finally, in a multicenter, long-term, randomized, placebo-controlled clinical trial, about 60% of MCI patients had reported some neuropsychiatric symptoms and almost half of the group had reported depressive symptoms (Feldman et al., 2004). Nonetheless, prevalence estimates of depressive symptoms in MCI had important limitations because it was impossible to establish a precise link between MCI and neuropsychiatric symptoms. Our present findings in conjunction with previous evidence (Jorm, 2000; Lyketsos et al., 2002; Chan et al., 2003; Forsell et al., 2003; Copeland et al., 2003; Hwang et al., 2004) suggest that depressive symptoms could be an early manifestation rather than a risk factor for MCI, arguing that the underlying pathology that causes MCI also causes depressive symptoms.

To the best of our knowledge, this is the first population-based study to report the incidence of depressive symptoms among patients with prevalent MCI. A prior non-population-based study of elderly volunteers estimated the incidence of depressive symptoms in MCI patients with a mean follow-up of 3.5 years to be 11.7 per 100 person-years (Li et al., 2001), that is less than half our incidence rate of depressive symptoms of 25.1 per 100 person-years, with a higher incidence of severe depressive symptoms (19.7 per 100 person-years). This underscores the importance of population-based studies, and the differences that may arise from selected groups. Finally, our findings suggest a borderline non-significant trend for a protective effect against the new-onset of total depressive symptoms in MCI subjects who reverted to normal cognition in comparison to cognitively stable MCI patients.

Current etiological models of late-life depression focus on the potential role of vascular risk factors, and suggest possible opportunities for specific prevention and intervention strategies in high-risk populations (Hickie and Scott, 1998; Prince et al., 1998), the so called "vascular depression" hypothesis (Alexopoulos et al., 1997; Krishnan et al., 1997). We failed to identify a possible impact of vascular disease or vascular risk factors on the onset of depressive symptoms in both cognitively stable MCI patients and in MCI patients who reverted to normal cognition after a 3.5 year follow-up. We found in a previous study a borderline trend of stroke as a risk factor of conversion of MCI to dementia (Solfrizzi et al., 2004), while stroke and cerebrovascular disease have been related to late-onset depression in several studies (Hickie and Scott, 1998; Prince et al., 1998; Kim et al., 2002). Nonetheless, in the present study stroke was not a risk factor for the onset of depressive symptoms in MCI patients. In fact, in cognitively normal subjects, the association of previous stroke with depressive symptoms was weaker in the presence of more severe cognitive impairment (Kim et al., 2002). Possibly, a follow-up period longer than 3.5 years would reveal that vascular risk factors could influence the onset of mood disturbances in MCI patients. Our findings were confirmed by a very recent prospective population-based study, the Leiden 85-Plus Study, in which vascular risk factors, and in particular generalized atherosclerosis, contributed to cognitive decline in old age but not to depression in a 3.3-year follow-up (Vinkers et al., 2005). In conclusion, given the complex interrelations among depressive symptoms, vascular risk factors, MCI, and dementia, further prospective studies with longer follow-up, measurements of depressive disorders, and vascular risk indicators early in the course of life are needed.

Depression and Risk of Predementia Syndromes

Converging evidence suggests that late-onset depressive symptoms or syndromes often are a prodrome of cognitive decline (Devanand et al., 1996; Bassuk et al., 1998; Yaffe et al.,

1999; Geerlings et al., 2000; Paterniti et al., 2002; Wilson et al., 2002; Fuhrer et al., 2003; Green et al., 2003; Wilson et al., 2004; Dal Forno et al., 2005; Gatz et al., 2005; Sachs-Ericsson et al., 2005; Barnes et al., 2006; Geda et al., 2006). Recent history of depression is associated with increased incidence of AD (Kokmen et al., 1991; Speck et al., 1995; Steffens et al., 1997). Individuals with late-life depression and transient cognitive impairment frequently develop AD or VaD within a few years after the onset of depression (Reding et al., 1985; Kral et al., 1989; Alexopoulos et al., 1993). Together, these observations suggest that some late-life depressive syndromes are early manifestations of dementing disorders. In contrast to the theory that depression represents a prodrome of dementia, there is growing evidence that depression may represent an independent risk factor predisposing to dementing disorders (Yaffe et al., 1999; Chen et al., 1999; Geerlings et al., 2000; Wilson et al., 2002; Green et al., 2003), even when depressive symptoms occur more than 10 years before the onset of dementia (Jorm et al., 1991; Speck et al., 1995). Lifetime history of depression increases the risk of AD, regardless of the presence or absence of family history of dementing disorders (van Duijn et al., 1994). Depression may be also a risk factor for VaD (Canadian Study of Health and Aging Working Group, 2000), and in depressed older adults with or without dementia, cognitive impairment may be related to the anticholinergic effects of medications prescribed or taken over the counter for depression or other conditions (Basu et al., 2003; Mulsant et al., 2003).

Our findings from the ILSA showed in a community defined Italian cohort, that higher depressive symptoms at baseline were not associated with the development of incident MCI or with the progression of MCI patients to dementia after a follow up at 3.5 years. No socio-demographic variables or vascular risk factors modified the association between depressive symptoms and incident MCI or between depressive symptoms and conversion to dementia (Panza etal., 2004). At present, only in the CHS Cognition Study the development of MCI was associated with measurements of cognition and depression (Lopez et al., 2003). Very recently, the CHS Cognition Study confirmed these findings in a prospective study with a 6-year follow-up, in which depressive symptoms at baseline were associated with increased risk of MCI and this association was independent of underlying vascular disease (Barnes et al., 2006). Finally, in a cohort of 840 cognitively normal elderly subjects without depression at recruitment who were followed-up prospectively for a median of 3.5 years, individuals in the depression cohort were at significantly increased risk of subsequent incident MCI, and a synergistic interaction between depression and APOE genotype was also found (Geda et al., 2006). These contrasting findings suggested that the length of the follow-period and the study design may be central for detecting an association between baseline depression and subsequent development of MCI. Our findings suggest that depression and MCI may co-occur, but fails to demonstrate a causal link between depressive symptoms and incident MCI, at least in a shorter follow-up. In fact, many recent studies determined among patients with MCI the prevalence of psychiatric symptoms, particularly anxiety and depression (Lyketsos et al., 2002; Chan et al., 2003; Forsell et al., 2003). A possible role of depressive symptoms was recently evaluated in preclinical AD (Berger et al., 1999; Visser et al., 2000), suggesting that depressive symptoms may be a part of the preclinical phase of dementia. Therefore, assuming that MCI may be the earliest identifiable clinical stage of dementia, the present findings confirm those of a large population based study showing that depressive symptoms may be an early manifestation rather than a risk factor for dementia and AD (Chen et al., 1999), arguing that the underlying pathology that causes MCI or dementia also causes depressive symptoms, rather than depressive symptoms causing or exacerbating MCI.

In the present population-based study, depressive symptoms failed to predict the conversion of MCI to dementia (Panza etal., 2004). Although some studies suggested a possible cluster between depressive symptoms and very mild cognitive impairment in predementia syndromes (Berger et al., 1999; Visser et al., 2000), depressive symptoms does not appear to be a risk factor for progression of MCI patients to dementia. Nonetheless, our findings are in contrast with those of another recent study in which patients with MCI and depression are at more than twice the risk of developing AD as those without depression after a mean period of 3 years (Modrego and Ferrandez, 2004). However, in this study a clinical diagnosis of depressive disorder was carried out, and the subjects were from a community general hospital and not from a population-based study. Furthermore, the results of the present report confirmed those of a recent study in which MCI patients who had concurrent depression did not have an increased risk of AD over two years compared to non-depressed MCI patients (Rozzini et al., 2005).

Previous studies have shown a correlation between vascular risk factors, such as hypertension, total cholesterol, and coronary artery disease and MCI (Di Carlo et al., 2000; DECarli et al., 2001; Solfrizzi et al., 2004; Panza et al., 2006a). Among subjects without coronary artery disease, the findings of the ILSA suggested that subjects with depressive symptoms should be at higher risk of incident MCI than those without depressive symptoms. However, when we adjusted for possible confounders, the predictive value of depressive symptoms for incident MCI in subjects without coronary artery disease was lost (Panza etal., 2004). Furthermore, we failed to find in our population a possible role of vascular risk factors on the depressive symptoms/dementia relationship. Possibly, a follow up longer than 3.5 years would reveal that vascular factors might influence the progression of MCI depressed patients to dementia. Among the socio-demographic factors estimated only gender modified the association between depressive symptoms and progression to dementia, with depressed women with MCI at higher risk for dementia, though we observed only a borderline non-significant effect (Panza etal., 2004).

Although our current findings did not suggest an effect of depressive symptoms on incident MCI or on the conversion of MCI to dementia, there is a considerable amount of evidence that depression can be associated with cognitive impairment in nondemented elderly people (Devanand et al., 1996; Bassuk et al., 1998; Yaffe et al., 1999; Geerlings et al., 2000; Paterniti et al., 2002; Wilson et al., 2002; Fuhrer et al., 2003; Green et al., 2003; Wilson et al., 2004; Dal Forno et al., 2005; Gatz et al., 2005; Sachs-Ericsson et al., 2005; Barnes et al., 2006; Geda et al., 2006). Contrasting findings about the impact of depressive symptoms on the development of MCI or cognitive dysfunction in normal elderly may suggest an approach not confined only to cognitive skills but extended to functional status and comorbidity. Therefore, a clinical diagnosis of MCI or dementia appeared to be cognitive outcomes more accurate in old age than neuropsychological testing only in order to study the temporal relationship between depression and cognitive impairment. Furthermore, socio-demographic variables and vascular risk factors did not seem to modify the relationships between depressive symptoms and incident MCI and between depressive symptoms and the progression to dementia in MCI patients. We found that only 2.2% of prevalent MCI patients used antidepressant drugs. This must reflect that subjects were not being adequately assessed and treated by their primary care clinicians, that higher depressive symptoms do not always translate into clinically significant depression, or both.

Depression and Predementia Syndromes: Possible Mechanisms

Some late-life depressive syndromes might predispose, precipitate, or perpetuate by CVD (Alexopoulos et al., 1997; Krishnan et al., 1997). This notion is based on the comorbidity of depressive syndromes with cerebrovascular lesions and cerebrovascular risk factors and on the fact that depression often develops after a stroke (Robinson, 2003). Elderly people with vascular depression have greater disability and cognitive impairment than those who are depressed but do not have vascular stigmata (Alexopoulos et al., 1997). Verbal fluency and object naming are the most impaired cognitive functions in patients with this form of depression. Affected individuals have more apathy, retardation, and lack of insight, and less agitation and guilt than do elderly individuals who are depressed without vascular risk factors (Alexopoulos et al., 1997; Krishnan et al., 1997). The vascular depression hypothesis generated hypotheses of clinical import. Drugs used for the prevention of CVD might, for example, reduce the risk for vascular depression. Furthermore, antidepressants that promote ischaemic recovery—eg, dopamine or norepinephrine enhancing agents—might be favoured in vascular depression and antidepressants that inhibit ischaemic recovery—eg, α adrenergic blocking agents—are best avoided (Alexopoulos et al., 1997). The possible association between depressive symptoms and MCI seems not attributable to vascular disease (Panza et al., 2004; Barnes et al., 2006), therefore there are several hypothesis on the underlying mechanism.

One hypothesis is that development of late-life depressive symptoms may reflect an underlying neuropathologic condition that manifests as cognitive decline over time. Therefore, depressive symptoms in the absence of overt cognitive impairment may reflect the early signs of a neurodegenerative disease. An alternative explanation is that the symptoms of depression may overlap to some extent with the symptoms of cognitive deterioration. Several other hypotheses may explain the relationship between depression and predementia syndromes. One possibility is that depression may be a causal factor, depression is in the chain of causality leading to MCI by virtue of its effect on the neuroendocrine axis (Sapolsky, 2001). An important implication of this hypothesis is that an intervention targeting depression may lead to primary prevention of MCI. Another hypothesis is that depression leads to damage in the hippocampus through a glucocorticoid cascade (Jorm, 2000; Jorm, 2001). This hypothesis is supported by research showing that older adults with high or rising cortisol levels during 5 years have poorer memory and greater hippocampal atrophy (Lupien et al., 1998).

Another possibility is that depression and predementia syndromes shared risk factor or confounding. In fact, depression is noncausally associated with MCI because a third factor leads to the genesis of both MCI and depression. The third factor (confounder) could be genetic, environmental, or both. A reverse causality is also possible, in fact, first, a person who is experiencing some degree of cognitive decline may develop depression as a reaction to the symptoms. Second, depressive symptoms may be an early noncognitive manifestation of dementia. Third, depression may "unmask" the clinical manifestations of MCI in individuals with limited cognitive reserve (Jorm et al., 1991). Another hypothesis is a possible interaction, in which depression leads to cognitive decline only in the presence of a genetic susceptibility factor or another risk factor. In fact, a very recent study found evidence of a synergistic interaction between APOE genotype and depression (Geda et al., 2006). There also may be a genetic link between depressive symptoms and dementia in some patients. For example, a study of women at high risk of carrying the presenilin 1 mutation for dementia showed that carriers of this mutation had significantly more depressive symptoms than noncarriers and were more likely to have sought help from a psychiatric professional (Ringman et al., 2004). All of these hypotheses, and perhaps others, await testing. Of course, these and other possible mechanisms are not mutually exclusive and may act in combination.

Conclusion

Recently, clinical research has focused on the identification of different clinical conditions that may represent a very early or preclinical symptomatic stage of dementing illnesses. Several studies have suggested that most of the patients who met the MCI criteria will progress to AD, but rates of conversion to AD and dementia vary widely among studies, partly because of the characteristics of the population involved and length of follow-up. Many of the risk factors for CVD and VaD have also been shown to increase the risk of AD. If MCI is essentially incipient AD, then factors predictive of AD should bear a similar relationship to MCI and both vascular factors and APOE ε4 allele have been associated with higher risk of AD. Nevertheless, recent evidence from a population-based study suggested that among MCI patients who progressed to dementia, 60% progressed to AD and 33% to VaD, reflecting the heterogeneity of MCI. Some recent studies further suggested that CVD or vascular factors increased risk of conversion from MCI to dementia. Although considerable epidemiological evidence indicates that cerebrovascular risk factors are associated with various types of dementia, including AD, only limited prospective information exists regarding the impact of CVD on incident dementia. Recent findings on the role of stroke in the progression of MCI to dementia, suggest a role of stroke and CVD in the natural history of predementia syndrome. Nevertheless, not all studies have shown an effect of CVD on the progression of MCI to dementia, suggesting that perhaps the main effect of cerebral infarction on the risk of post-stroke cognitive impairment is when the infarction itself causes it.

The amnestic form of MCI has received considerable research attention, but much less is known about the nonamnestic subtypes. Additional research is needed to describe the neuropsychological, neuropathological, and neuroradiological characteristics and progression of each of the suggested subtypes and to identify factors that predict progression, with specific attention to the role of depression. The critical question is how the presence of depression modifies the risk of progression from MCI to dementia. Studies that refine our knowledge about the subtypes of MCI and cognitive decline and about the role of depression in them will also have an effect on our clinical and research diagnostic nomenclature and conceptualization of illness. Longitudinal studies can compare the predictive validity for outcomes of the different subtypes. Specifically, research is needed to clarify whether mood symptoms might be included in diagnostic criteria sets, act as a modifier, be excluded from the MCI diagnosis, or be seen as 1 of 2 distinct but not mutually exclusive diagnoses (Steffens et al., 2006).

Clinical presentations of depression in old age have considerable variability, suggesting the need for a broad approach to assessment of co-occurring depression and cognitive impairment. The approach should be adequate for capturing the range of depressive symptoms and behavioral manifestations that occur in the context of cognitive impairment, especially those that occur in the early stages of impairment. Other areas that should be assessed might include personality, appetite changes, sleep apnea and other sleep disturbances, as well as childhood traumatic events, depression history, and other background characteristics that could predict ultimate cognitive impairment (Steffens et al., 2006).

Specific cognitive impairments and the putative underlying neurobiological disturbances determine not only the course of cognitive impairment but also the course of affective impairment. Additional studies are needed to follow up on the implications of these findings to understand the mechanisms linking depression and dementia and to identify other biomarkers. The most consistent findings are structural measures (eg, regional atrophy and mediotemporal atrophy), positron emission tomography functional measures, and several promising cerebrospinal fluid measures. APOE genotype is the most consistent genetic marker, but others are being examined. Future research will need to reconcile the seemingly divergent paths of research regarding the underlying pathologic features that are seen on neuroimaging. Postmortem evaluations for neuropathologic conditions are needed to further understand disease mechanisms and biomarkers (Sweet et al., 2004). Other types of specimens should be banked so that they will be available for later use when additional reliable biomarkers are identified.

Acknowledgements

This group is supported by Italian Longitudinal Study on Aging (ILSA) (Italian National Research Council - CNR-Targeted Project on Ageing - Grants 9400419PF40 and 95973PF40), by AFORIGE ("Associazione per la FOrmazione e la RIcerca in Geriatria"). The authors thank Dr Luciana Lacriola and for her assistance with bibliographic sources and for editing the manuscript. Conflict of interest: none declared

References

American Psychiatric Association Committee on Nomenclature and Statistics. *Diagnostic and Statistical Manual of Mental Disorders*. 3rd Edition revised (DSM-III-R). American Psychiatric Association, Washington, DC, 1987.

American Psychiatric Association Committee on Nomenclature and Statistics. *Diagnostic and Statistical Manual of Mental Disorders*. 4th Edition (DSM-IV). American Psychiatric Association, Washington, DC, 1994.

Ancelin ML, Artero S, Portet F, Dupuy AM, Touchon J, Ritchie K. Non-degenerative mild cognitive impairment in elderly people and use of anticholinergic drugs: longitudinal cohort study. *BMJ*. 2006;332(7539):455-459.

Alexopoulos GS, Meyers BS, Young RC, Mattis S, Kakuma T. The course of geriatric depression with "reversible dementia": a controlled study. *Am. J. Psychiatry* 1993;150:1693-1699.

Alexopoulos GS, Meyers BS, Young RC, Kakuma T, Silbersweig D, Charlson M. Clinically defined vascular depression. *Am. J. Psychiatry* 1997;154:562-565.

Alexopoulos GS, Buckwalter K, Olin J, Martinez R, Wainscott C, Krishnan KR. Comorbidity of late-life depression: an opportunity for research in mechanisms and treatment. *Biol. Psychiatry* 2002; 52:543–558.

Alexopoulos GS. Depression in the elderly. *Lancet* 2005;365:1961-1970.

Andersen K, Lolk A, Nielsen H, Andersen J, Olsen C, Kragh-Sorensen P. Prevalence of very mild to severe dementia in Denmark. *Acta Neurol Scand* 1997;96:82-87.

Andersen K, Nielsen H, Lolk A, Andersen J, Becker I, Kragh-Sorensen P. Incidence of very mild to severe dementia and Alzheimer's disease in Denmark: the Odense Study. *Neurology* 1999;52:85-90.

Asberg M, Montgomery SA, Perris C, Schalling D, Sedvall G. A comprehensive psychopathological rating scale. *Acta Psychiatr Scand Suppl.* 1978;271:5-27.

Bassuk SS, Berkman LF, Wypij D. Depressive symptomatology and incident cognitive decline in an elderly community sample. *Arch. Gen. Psychiatry* 1998;55:1073-1081.

Basu R, Dodge H, Stoehr GP, Ganguli M. Sedative-hypnotic use of diphenhydramine in a rural, older adult, community-based cohort: effects on cognition. *Am. J. Geriatr. Psychiatry* 2003;11:205-213.

Barnes DE, Alexopoulos GS, Lopez OL, Williamson JD, Yaffe K. Depressive symptoms, vascular disease, and mild cognitive impairment: findings from the Cardiovascular Health Study. *Arch. Gen. Psychiatry* 2006;63:273-279.

Berger AK, Fratiglioni L, Forsell Y, Winblad B, Backman L. The occurrence of depressive symptoms in the preclinical phase of AD: a population-based study. *Neurology* 1999;53:1998-2002.

Blackford RC, La Rue A. Criteria for diagnosing age-associated memory impairment: proposed improvements from the field. *Dev. Neuropsychol* 1989;5:295-306

Blazer DG. Depression in late life: review and commentary. *J. Gerontol Med Sci* 2003;56A: 249–265.

Bischkopf J, Busse A, Angermeyer MC. Mild cognitive impairment--a review of prevalence, incidence and outcome according to current approaches. *Acta. Psychiatr. Scand.* 2002;106:403-414.

Blair CK, Folsom AR, Knopman DS, Bray MS, Mosley TH, Boerwinkle E; Atherosclerosis Risk in Communities (ARIC) Study Investigators.. APOE genotype and cognitive decline in a middle-aged cohort. *Neurology* 2005; 64: 268-276.

Bozoki A, Giordani B, Heidebrink JL, Berent S, Foster NL. Mild cognitive impairments predict dementia in nondemented elderly patients with memory loss. *Arch. Neurol.* 2001;58:411–416.

Busse A, Bischkopf J, Riedel-Heller SG, Angermeyer MC. Subclassifications for mild cognitive impairment: prevalence and predictive validity. *Psychol. Med.* 2003;33:1029-1038.

Chan DC, Kasper JD, Black BS, Rabins PV. Prevalence and correlates of behavioral and psychiatric symptoms in community-dwelling elders with dementia or mild cognitive impairment: the Memory and Medical Care Study. *Int. J. Geriatr Psychiatry* 2003;18:174-182.

Charney DS, Reynolds CF 3rd, Lewis L, Lebowitz BD, Sunderland T, Alexopoulos GS, Blazer DG, Katz IR, Meyers BS, Arean PA, Borson S, Brown C, Bruce ML, Callahan CM, Charlson ME, Conwell Y, Cuthbert BN, Devanand DP, Gibson MJ, Gottlieb GL, Krishnan KR, Laden SK, Lyketsos CG, Mulsant BH, Niederehe G, Olin JT, Oslin DW, Pearson J, Persky T, Pollock BG, Raetzman S, Reynolds M, Salzman C, Schulz R, Schwenk TL, Scolnick E, Unutzer J, Weissman MM, Young RC; Depression and Bipolar Support Alliance. Depression and Bipolar Support Alliance consensus statement on the unmet needs in diagnosis and treatment of mood disorders in late life. *Arch. Gen. Psychiatry* 2003; 60: 664–672.

Canadian Study of Health and Aging Working Group. The incidence of dementia in Canada. *Neurology* 2000;55:66-73.

Chen P, Ganguli M, Mulsant BH, DeKosky ST. The temporal relationship between depressive symptoms and dementia: a community-based prospective study. *Arch. Gen. Psychiatry* 1999;56:261-266.

Christensen H, Henderson AS, Jorm AF, Mackinnon AJ, Scott R, Korten AE. ICD-10 mild cognitive disorder: epidemiological evidence on its validity. *Psychol. Med.* 1995;25:105-120.

Copeland MP, Daly E, Hines V, Mastromauro C, Zaitchik D, Gunther J, Albert M. Psychiatric symptomatology and prodromal Alzheimer's disease. *Alzheimer Dis. Assoc. Disord.* 2003;17:1-8.

Crook T, Bartus RT, Ferris SH, Whitehouse P, Cohen GD, Gershon S. Age associated memory impairment: proposed diagnostic criteria and measures of clinical change-report of a National Institute of Mental Health work group. *Dev. Neuropsychol.* 1986;2:261-276

Cummings JL, Mega M, Gray K, Rosenberg-Thompson S, Carusi DA, Gornbein J. The Neuropsychiatric Inventory: comprehensive assessment of psychopathology in dementia. *Neurology* 1994;44:2308-2314.

Dal Forno G, Palermo MT, Donohue JE, Karagiozis H, Zonderman AB, Kawas CH. Depressive symptoms, sex, and risk for Alzheimer's disease. *Ann. Neurol.* 2005;57:381-387.

DeCarli C, Miller BL, Swan GE, Reed T, Wolf PA, Carmelli D. Cerebrovascular and brain morphologic correlates of mild cognitive impairment in the National Heart, Lung, and Blood Institute Twin Study. *Arch. Neurol.* 2001;58:643–647.

Devanand DP, Sano M, Tang MX, Taylor S, Gurland BJ, Wilder D, Stern Y, Mayeux R. Depressed mood and the incidence of Alzheimer's disease in the elderly living in the community. *Arch. Gen. Psychiatry* 1996;53:175-182.

DeCarli C, Mungas D, Harvey D, Reed B, Weiner M, Chui H, Jagust W. Memory impairment, but not cerebrovascular disease, predicts progression of MCI to dementia. *Neurology* 2004;63:220–227.

Di Carlo A, Baldereschi M, Amaducci L, Maggi S, Grigoletto F, Scarlato G, Inzitari D. Cognitive impairment without dementia in older people: prevalence, vascular risk factors, impact on disability. The Italian Longitudinal Study on Aging. *J. Am. Geriatr. Soc.* 2000;48:775-782.

D'Introno A, Panza F, Colacicco AM, Capurso A, Solfrizzi V. Mild Cognitive Impairment and related entities: role of vascular risk factors. In: Panza, F; Solfrizzi, V; Capurso, A. *Diet and Cognitive Decline*. NY, USA: Nova Science Publishers, Inc; 2004; pp 1-33.

Dik MG, Jonker C, Bouter LM, Geerlings MI, van Kamp GJ, Deeg DJ. APOE-epsilon4 is associated with memory decline in cognitively impaired elderly. *Neurology* 2000;54: 1492-1497.

Dubois B, Albert ML. Amnestic MCI or prodromal Alzheimer's disease? *Lancet Neurol.* 2004;3:246-248.

Dufouil C, Fuhrer R, Dartigues JF, Alperovitch A. Longitudinal analysis of the association between depressive symptomatology and cognitive deterioration. *Am J. Epidemiol.* 1996;144:634-641.

Ebly EM, Parhad IM, Hogan DB, Fung TS. Prevalence and types of dementia in the very old: results from the Canadian Study of Health and Aging. *Neurology* 1994;44:1593-1600.

Ebly EM, Hogan DB, Parhad IM. Cognitive impairment in the nondemented elderly. Results from the Canadian Study of Health and Aging. *Arch. Neurol.* 1995;52:612-619.

Feldman H, Scheltens P, Scarpini E, Hermann N, Mesenbrink P, Mancione L, Tekin S, Lane R, Ferris S. Behavioral symptoms in mild cognitive impairment. *Neurology* 2004;62:1199-1201.

Frisoni GB, Galluzzi S, Bresciani L, Zanetti O, Geroldi C. Mild cognitive impairment with subcortical vascular features: clinical characteristics and outcome. *J. Neurol.* 2002;249:1423-1432.

First MB, Spitzer RL, Gibbon M, Williams JBW. *Structured Clinical Interview for DSM-IV Axis I Disorders (SCID I)*, Clinician Version, Administration Booklet. Washington, DC: American Psychiatric Press; 1997.

Flicker C, Ferris SH, Reisberg B. Mild cognitive impairment in the elderly: predictors of dementia. *Neurology* 1991;41:1006–1009.

Forsell Y, Palmer K, Fratiglioni L. Psychiatric symptoms/syndromes in elderly persons with mild cognitive impairment. Data from a cross-sectional study. *Acta. Neurol. Scand. Suppl.* 2003;179:25-28.

Frisoni GB, Galluzzi S, Bresciani L, Zanetti O, Geroldi C. Mild cognitive impairment with subcortical vascular features: clinical characteristics and outcome. *J. Neurol.* 2002;249:1423-1432.

Fuhrer R, Dufouil C, Dartigues JF; PAQUID Study. Exploring sex differences in the relationship between depressive symptoms and dementia incidence: prospective results from the PAQUID Study. *J. Am. Geriatr. Soc.* 2003;51:1055-1063.

Gallo JJ, Rabins PV, Lyketsos LG, Tien AY, Anthony JC. Depression without sadness: functional outcomes of nondysphoric depression in later life. *J. Am. Geriatr. Soc.* 1997;45:570-578.

Ganguli M, Dodge HH, Shen C, DeKosky ST. Mild cognitive impairment, amnestic type: an epidemiologic study. *Neurology* 2004;63:115-121.

Ganguli M, Du Y, Dodge HH, Ratcliff GG, Chang CC. Depressive symptoms and cognitive decline in late life: a prospective epidemiological study. *Arch. Gen. Psychiatry* 2006;63:153-160.

Gauthier S, Touchon J. Mild cognitive impairment is not a clinical entity and should not be treated. *Arch. Neurol.* 2005;62:1164-1166.

Gauthier S, Reisberg B, Zaudig M, Petersen RC, Ritchie K, Broich K, Belleville S, Brodaty H, Bennett D, Chertkow H, Cummings JL, de Leon M, Feldman H, Ganguli M, Hampel H, Scheltens P, Tierney MC, Whitehouse P, Winblad B; International Psychogeriatric Association Expert Conference on mild cognitive impairment. Mild cognitive impairment. *Lancet* 2006;367:1262-1270.

Gatz JL, Tyas SL, St John P, Montgomery P. Do depressive symptoms predict Alzheimer's disease and dementia? *J. Gerontol A Biol. Sci. Med. Sci.* 2005;60:744-747.

Geda YE, Smith GE, Knopman DS, Boeve BF, Tangalos EG, Ivnik RJ, Mrazek DA, Edland SD, Petersen RC. De novo genesis of neuropsychiatric symptoms in mild cognitive impairment. *Int. Psychogeriatr.* 2004;16:51-60.

Geda YE, Knopman DS, Mrazek DA, Jicha GA, Smith GE, Negash S, Boeve BF, Ivnik RJ, Petersen RC, Pankratz VS, Rocca WA. Depression, apolipoprotein E genotype, and the incidence of mild cognitive impairment: a prospective cohort study. *Arch. Neurol.* 2006;63:435-440.

Geerlings MI, Schoevers RA, Beekman AT, Jonker C, Deeg DJ, Schmand B, Ader HJ, Bouter LM, Van Tilburg W. Depression and risk of cognitive decline and Alzheimer's disease. Results of two prospective community-based studies in The Netherlands. *Br. J. Psychiatry* 2000;176:568-575.

Goldman WP, Price JL, Storandt M, Grant EA, McKeel DW Jr, Rubin EH, Morris JC. Absence of cognitive impairment or decline in preclinical Alzheimer's disease. *Neurology*. 2001;56:361-367.

Green RC, Cupples LA, Kurz A, Auerbach S, Go R, Sadovnick D, Duara R, Kukull WA, Chui H, Edeki T, Griffith PA, Friedland RP, Bachman D, Farrer L. Depression as a risk factor for Alzheimer disease: the MIRAGE Study. *Arch. Neurol.* 2003;60:753-759.

Gurland BJ, Dean LL, Copeland J. Criteria for diagnosis of dementia in the community elderly. *Gerontologist* 1982;22:180-186.

Henon H, Durieu I, Guerouaou D, Lebert F, Pasquier F, Leys D. Poststroke dementia: incidence and relationship to prestroke cognitive decline. *Neurology* 2001;57:1216-1212.

Hogan DB, McKeith IG: Of MCI and dementia: improving diagnosis and treatment. *Neurology* 2001;56:1131-1132.

Hickie I, Scott E. Late-onset depressive disorders: a preventable variant of cerebrovascular disease? *Psycho.l Med.* 1998;28:1007-1013.

Holtzer R, Scarmeas N, Wegesin DJ, Albert M, Brandt J, Dubois B, Hadjigeorgiou GM, Stern Y. Depressive symptoms in Alzheimer's disease: natural course and temporal relation to function and cognitive status. *J. Am. Geriatr. Soc.* 2005;53:2083-2089.

Hughes CP, Berg L, Danziger WL, Coben LA, Martin RL. A new clinical scale for the staging of dementia. *Br. J. Psychiatry* 1982;140: 566-572.

Hwang TJ, Masterman DL, Ortiz F, Fairbanks LA, Cummings JL. Mild cognitive impairment is associated with characteristic neuropsychiatric symptoms. *Alzheimer Dis. Assoc. Disord.* 2004;18:17-21.

Jonker C, Schmand B, Lindeboom J, Havekes LM, Launer LJ. Association between apolipoprotein E epsilon4 and the rate of cognitive decline in community-dwelling elderly individuals with and without dementia. *Arch. Neuro.l* 1998;55:1065-1069.

Jorm AF, van Duijn CM, Chandra V, Fratiglioni L, Graves AB, Heyman A, Kokmen E, Kondo K, Mortimer JA, and Rocca WA; EURODEM Risk Factors Research Group. Psychiatric history and related exposures as risk factors for Alzheimer's disease: a collaborative re-analysis of case-control studies. *Int. J. Epidemiol.* 1991;20(Suppl 2):S43-S47.

Jorm AF. Is depression a risk factor for dementia or cognitive decline? *Gerontology* 2000;46:219-227.

Jorm AF. History of depression as a risk factor for dementia: an updated review. *Aust N Z J Psychiatry* 2001;35:776-781.

Kim JM, Stewart R, Shin IS, Yoon JS. Previous stroke but not vascular risk factors are associated with depression in a cognitively impaired older Korean population. *Int. J. Geriatr. Psychiatry* 2002;17:453-458.

Kivipelto M, Helkala EL, Hanninen T, Laakso MP, Hallikainen M, Alhainen K, Soininen H, Tuomilehto J, Nissinen A. Midlife vascular risk factors and late-life mild cognitive impairment. A population-based study. *Neurology* 2001a;56:1683-1689.

Kivipelto M, Helkala EL, Laakso MP, Hanninen T, Hallikainen M, Alhainen K, Soininen H, Tuomilehto J, Nissinen A. Midlife vascular risk factors and Alzheimer's disease in later life: longitudinal, population based study. *BMJ* 2001b;322:1447–1451.

Kokmen E, Beard CM, Chandra V, Offord KP, Schoenberg BS, Ballard DJ. Clinical risk factors for Alzheimer's disease: a population-based case-control study. *Neurology* 1991;41:1393-1397.

Kral VA. Senescent forgetfulness: benign and malignant. *Can. Med. Assoc. J.* 1962;86:257-260.

Kral VA, Emery OB. Long-term follow-up of depressive pseudodementia of the aged. *Can. J. Psychiatry* 1989;34:445-446.

Krishnan KR, Hays JC, Blazer DG. MRI-defined vascular depression. *Am. J. Psychiatry* 1997;154:497-501.

Larrieu S, Letenneur L, Orgogozo JM, Fabrigoule C, Amieva H, Le Carret N, Barberger-Gateau P, Dartigues JF. Incidence and outcome of mild cognitive impairment in a population-based prospective cohort. *Neurology* 2002;59:1594-1599.

Larson EB. Illnesses causing dementia in the very elderly. *N. Engl. J. Med* .1993;328:203-205.

Levy R. Aging-associated cognitive decline. Working Party of the International Psychogeriatric Association in collaboration with the World Health Organization. *Int. Psychogeriatrics* 1994;6:63-68.

Li YS, Meyer JS, Thornby J. Longitudinal follow-up of depressive symptoms among normal versus cognitively impaired elderly. *Int J. Geriatr. Psychiatry* 2001;16:718-727.

Linn RT, Wolf PA, Bachman DL, Knoefel JE, Cobb JL, Belanger AJ, Kaplan EF, D'Agostino RB. The 'preclinical phase' of probable Alzheimer's disease. A 13-year prospective study of the Framingham cohort. *Arch. Neurol.* 1995;52:485-490.

Lopez OL, Jagust WJ, Dulberg C, Becker JT, DeKosky ST, Fitzpatrick A, Breitner J, Lyketsos C, Jones B, Kawas C, Carlson M, Kuller LH. Risk factors for mild cognitive impairment in the cardiovascular health study cognition study: part 2. *Arch. Neurol.* 2003;60:1394–1399.

Luis CA, Loewenstein DA, Acevedo A, Barker WW, Duara R. Mild cognitive impairment: directions for future research. *Neurology* 2003;61:438-444.

Lupien SJ, de Leon M, de Santi S, Convit A, Tarshish C, Nair NP, Thakur M, McEwen BS, Hauger RL, Meaney MJ. Cortisol levels during human aging predict hippocampal atrophy and memory deficits. *Nat Neurosci.* 1998;1:69-73.

Lyketsos CG, Lopez O, Jones B, Fitzpatrick AL, Breitner J, DeKosky S. Prevalence of neuropsychiatric symptoms in dementia and mild cognitive impairment: results from the cardiovascular health study. *JAMA* 2002;288:1475-1483.

Lyness JM, King DA, Cox C, Yoediono Z, Caine ED. The importance of subsyndromal depression in older primary care patients: prevalence and associated functional disability. *J. Am.Geriatr. Soc.* 1999;47:647-652.

Manly JJ, Bell-McGinty S, Tang MX, Schupf N, Stern Y, Mayeux R. Implementing diagnostic criteria and estimating frequency of mild cognitive impairment in an urban community. *Arch. Neurol.* 2005;62:1739-1746.

Modrego PJ, Ferrandez J. Depression in patients with mild cognitive impairment increases the risk of developing dementia of Alzheimer type: a prospective cohort study. *Arch. Neurol.* 2004;61:1290-1293.

Morris JC, Edland S, Clark C, Galasko D, Koss E, Mohs R, van Belle G, Fillenbaum G, Heyman A. The consortium to establish a registry for Alzheimer's disease (CERAD). Part IV. Rates of cognitive change in the longitudinal assessment of probable Alzheimer's disease. *Neurology* 1993;43:2457-2465.

Morris JC, Storandt M, Miller JP, McKeel DW, Price JL, Rubin EH, Berg L. Mild cognitive impairment represents early-stage Alzheimer disease. *Arch. Neurol.* 2001;58:397-405.

Mulsant BH, Pollock BG, Kirshner M, Shen C, Dodge HH, Ganguli M. Serum anticholinergic activity in a community-based sample of older adults. *Arch. Gen. Psychiatry* 2003;60:198-203.

Neuropathology Group of the Medical Research Council Cognitive Function and Ageing Study (MRC CFAS). Pathological correlates of late-onset dementia in a multicentre, community-based population in England and Wales. *Lancet* 2001;357:169-175.

Olin JT, Schneider LS, Katz IR, Meyers BS, Alexopoulos GS, Breitner JC, Bruce ML, Caine ED, Cummings JL, Devanand DP, Krishnan KR, Lyketsos CG, Lyness JM, Rabins PV, Reynolds CF 3rd, Rovner BW, Steffens DC, Tariot PN, Lebowitz BD. Provisional diagnostic criteria for depression of Alzheimer's disease. *Am. J. Geriatr. Psychiatry* 2002; 10: 125–28.

Palsson S, Aevarsson O, Skoog I. Depression, cerebral atrophy, cognitive performance and incidence of dementia. Population study of 85-year-olds. *Br. J. Psychiatry* 1999;174:249-253.

Panza F, D'Introno A, Colacicco AM, Basile AM, Capurso C, Kehoe PG, et al. Vascular risk and genetics of sporadic late-onset Alzheimer's disease. *J. Neural Transm.* 2004;111:69-89.

Panza F, Solfrizzi V, D'Introno A, Colacicco AM, Capurso C, Torres F, Pellicani V, Capurso A.Mild Cognitive Impairment, demenza e sintomatologia depressiva: rapporti di contiguità e continuità. *Dementia Update* 2004;17: 15-25.

Panza F, D'Introno A, Colacicco AM, Capurso C, Del Parigi A, Caselli RJ, Pilotto A, Argentieri G, Scapicchio PL, Scafato E, Capurso A, Solfrizzi V. Current epidemiology of mild cognitive impairment and other predementia syndromes. *Am. J. Geriatr. Psychiatry* 2005;13:633-644.

Panza F, D'Introno A, Colacicco AM, Capurso C, Parigi AD, Capurso SA, Caselli RJ, Pilotto A, Scafato E, Capurso A, Solfrizzi V. Cognitive frailty: Predementia syndrome and vascular risk factors. *Neurobiol. Aging* 2006a;27:933-940.

Panza F, D'Introno A, Colacicco AM, Capurso C, Parigi AD, Capurso A, Solfrizzi V. Heterogeneity of mild cognitive impairment and other predementia syndromes in progression to dementia. *Neurobiol Aging* 2006b: doi:10.1016 /j.neurobiolaging. 2006.07.019.

Panza F, Capurso C, D'Introno A, Colacicco AM, Capurso A, Solfrizzi V. Prevalence rates of mild cognitive impairment subtypes and progression to dementia. *J. Am. Geriatr.Soc.* 2006c;54:1474-475.

Panza F, Capurso C, D'Introno A, Colacicco AM, Capurso A, Solfrizzi V. Mild cognitive impairment: risk of Alzheimer disease and rate of cognitive decline. *Neurology* 2006d (in press).

Panza F, Solfrizzi V, Colacicco AM, D'Introno A, Capurso C, Palasciano R, Todarello O, Capurso S, Pellicani V, Capurso A. Cerebrovascular disease in the elderly: lipoprotein metabolism and cognitive decline. *Aging Clin. Exp. Res.* 2006e;18:144-148.

Paterniti S, Verdier-Taillefer MH, Dufouil C, Alperovitch A. Depressive symptoms and cognitive decline in elderly people. Longitudinal study. *Br. J. Psychiatry* 2002;181:406-410.

Petersen RC, Smith GE, Ivnik RJ, Tangalos EG, Schaid DJ, Thibodeau SN, Kokmen E, Waring SC, Kurland LT. Apolipoprotein E status as a predictor of the development of Alzheimer's disease in memory-impaired individuals. *JAMA* 1995;273:1274–1278.

Petersen RC, Waring SC, Smith GE, Tangalos EG, Thibodeau SN. Predictive value of APOE genotyping in incipient Alzheimer's disease. *Ann. NY Acad. Sci.*1996;802:58–69.

Petersen RC, Smith GE, Waring SC, Ivnik RJ, Tangalos EG, Kokmen E. Mild cognitive impairment: clinical characterization and outcome. *Arch. Neurol.* 1999;56:303-308.

Petersen RC, Stevens JC, Ganguli M, Tangalos EG, Cummings JL, DeKosky ST. Practice parameter: early detection of dementia: mild cognitive impairment (an evidence-based review). Report of the Quality Standards Subcommittee of the American Academy of Neurology. *Neurology* 2001a;56:1133-1142

Petersen RC, Doody R, Kurz A, et al: Current concepts in mild cognitive decline. Ar*ch. Neurol.* 2001b;58:1985-1992.

Portet F, Ousset PJ, Visser PJ, Frisoni GB, Nobili F, Scheltens P, Vellas B, Touchon J; MCI Working Group of the European Consortium on Alzheimer's Disease (EADC). Mild cognitive impairment (MCI) in medical practice: a critical review of the concept and new diagnostic procedure. Report of the MCI Working Group of the European Consortium on Alzheimer's Disease. *J. Neurol. Neurosurg. Psychiatry* 2006;77:714-718.

Prince MJ, Harwood RH, Thomas A, Mann AH. A prospective population-based cohort study of the effects of disablement and social milieu on the onset and maintenance of late-life depression. The Gospek Oak Project VII. *Psychol. Med.* 1998;8:337-350.

Orsitto G, Seripa D, Panza F, Franceschi M, Cascavilla L, Placentino G, Matera MG, Paris F, Solfrizzi V, Dallapiccola B, Pilotto A. Apolipoprotein E genotypes in mild cognitive impairment subtypes. *J. Am. Geriatr .Soc* .2006;54:1965-1966.

Rediess S, Caine ED. Aging, cognition, and DSM-IV. Aging, *Neuropsychology, Cognition* 1996;3:105-117.

Reding M, Haycox J, Blass J. Depression in patients referred to a dementia clinic: a three-year prospective study. *Arch. Neurol.* 1985;42:894-896.

Reisberg B, Ferris SH, de Leon MJ, Crook T. The Global Deterioration Scale for assessment of primary degenerative dementia. *Am. J. Psychiatry.* 1982;139: 1136-1139.

Riley KP, Snowdon DA, Markesbery WR. Alzheimer's neurofibrillary pathology and the spectrum of cognitive function: findings from the Nun Study. Ann Neurol 2002;51:567–577.

Ringman JM, Diaz-Olavarrieta C, Rodriguez Y, Chavez M, Paz F, Murrell J, Macias MA, Hill M, Kawas C. Female preclinical presenilin-1 mutation carriers unaware of their genetic status have higher levels of depression than their nonmutation carrying kin. *J. Neurol Neurosurg. Psychiatry.* 2004;75:500-502.

Robinson RG. Poststroke depression: prevalence, diagnosis, treatment, and disease prevention. *Biol. Psychiatry* 2003; 54: 376–387.

Romas SN, Tang MX, Berglund L, Mayeux R. APOE genotype, plasma lipids, lipoproteins, and AD in community elderly. *Neurology* 1999;53:517-521.

Roth M, Tym E, Mountjoy CQ, Huppert FA, Hendrie H, Verma S, Goddard R. CAMDEX. A standardized instrument for the diagnosis of mental disorder in the elderly with special reference to the early detection of dementia. *Br. J. Psychiatry* 1986;149: 698-709

Rozzini L, Chilovi BV, Trabucchi M, Padovani A. Depression is unrelated to conversion to dementia in patients with mild cognitive impairment. *Arch. Neurol.* 2005;62:505.

Sachs-Ericsson N, Joiner T, Plant EA, Blazer DG. The influence of depression on cognitive decline in community-dwelling elderly persons. *Am. J. Geriatr. Psychiatry* 2005;13:402-408.

Sapolsky RM. Depression, antidepressants, and the shrinking hippocampus. *Proc. Natl. Acad. Sci. USA* 2001;98:12320-12322.

Schneider JA, Wilson RS, Bienias JL, Evans DA, Bennett DA. Cerebral infarctions and the likelihood of dementia from Alzheimer disease pathology. *Neurology* 2004;62:1148-1155.

Small BJ, Basun H, Backman L. Three-year changes in cognitive performance as a function of apolipoprotein E genotype: evidence from very old adults without dementia. *Psychol. Aging* 1998;13: 80-87.

Sobin C, Sacheim HA. Psychomotor symptoms of depression. *Am. J. Psychiatry* 1997; 154: 4–17.

Solfrizzi V, Panza F, Torres F, Mastroianni F, Del Parigi A, Venezia A, Capurso A. High monounsaturated fatty acids intake protects against age-related cognitive decline. *Neurology* 1999;52:1524-1530.

Solfrizzi V, Panza F, D'Introno A, Colacicco AM, Capurso C, Basile AM, Capurso A. Lipoprotein(a), apolipoprotein E genotype, and risk of Alzheimer's disease. *J. Neurol. Neurosurg. Psychiatry* 2002;72:732-736.

Solfrizzi V, Panza F, Capurso A. The role of diet in cognitive decline. *J. Neural Transm.* 2003;110:95-110.

Solfrizzi V, Panza F, Colacicco AM, D'Introno A, Capurso C, Torres F, Grigoletto F, Maggi S, Del Parigi A, Reiman EM, Caselli RJ, Scafato E, Farchi G, Capurso A; Italian Longitudinal Study on Aging Working Group. Vascular risk factors, incidence of MCI, and rates of progression to dementia. *Neurology* 2004;63:1882-1891.

Speck CE, Kukull WA, Brenner DE, Bowen JD, McCormick WC, Teri L, Peterson G, Hooton TM, Collier AC, Corey L, Koutsky L, Krieger JN. History of depression as a risk factor for Alzheimer's disease. *Epidemiology* 1995;6:366-369.

Srikanth VK, Anderson JF, Donnan GA, Saling MM, Didus E, Alpitsis R, Dewey HM, Macdonell RA, Thrift AG. Progressive dementia after first-ever stroke. A community-based follow-up study. *Neurology* 2004;63:785-792.

Steffens DC, Plassman BL, Helms MJ, Welsh-Bohmer KA, Saunders AM, Breitner JC. A twin study of late-onset depression and apolipoprotein E ε4 as risk factors for Alzheimer's disease. *Biol. Psychiatry* 1997;41:851-856

Steffens DC, Otey E, Alexopoulos GS, Butters MA, Cuthbert B, Ganguli M, Geda YE, Hendrie HC, Krishnan RR, Kumar A, Lopez OL, Lyketsos CG, Mast BT, Morris JC, Norton MC, Peavy GM, Petersen RC, Reynolds CF, Salloway S, Welsh-Bohmer KA, Yesavage J. Perspectives on depression, mild cognitive impairment, and cognitive decline. *Arch. Gen. Psychiatry* 2006;63:130-138.

Sweet RA, Hamilton RL, Butters MA, Mulsant BH, Bollock BG, Lewis DA, DeKosky ST, Reynolds CF. Neuropathology correlates of late-onset major depression. *Neuropsychopharmacology.* 2004;29:2242-2250.

Tervo S, Kivipelto M, Hanninen T, Vanhanen M, Hallikainen M, Mannermaa A, Soininen H. Incidence and risk factors for mild cognitive impairment: a population-based three-year follow-up study of cognitively healthy elderly subjects. *Dement Geriatr. Cogn. Disord.* 2004;17:196-203.

Traykov L, Rigaud AS, Baudic S, Smagghe A, Boller F, Forette F. Apolipoprotein E epsilon 4 allele frequency in demented and cognitively impaired patients with and without cerebrovascular disease. *J. Neurol. Sci.* 2002;203/204: 177-181.

van Duijn CM, Clayton DG, Chandra V, Fratiglioni L, Graves AB, Heyman A, Jorm AF, Kokmen E, Kondo K, Mortimer JA. Interaction between genetic and environmental risk factors for Alzheimer's disease: a reanalysis of case-control studies. *Genet. Epidemiol.* 1994;11:539-551.

Vermeer SE, Prins ND, den Heijer T, Hofman A, Koudstaal PJ, Breteler MM. Silent brain infarcts and the risk of dementia and cognitive decline. *N. Engl. J. Med.* 2003;348:1215–1222.

Visser PJ, Verhey FR, Ponds RW, Kester A, Jolles J. Distinction between preclinical Alzheimer's disease and depression. *J. Am. Geriatr. Soc.* 2000;48:479-484.

Vinkers DJ, Gussekloo J, Stek ML, et al. Temporal relation between depression and cognitive impairment in old age: prospective population based study. *BMJ* 2004;329:881.

Vinkers DJ, Stek ML, van der Mast RC, de Craen AJ, Le Cessie S, Jolles J, Westendorp RG, Gussekloo J. Generalized atherosclerosis, cognitive decline, and depressive symptoms in old age. *Neurology* 2005;65:107-212.

Zanetti M, Ballabio C, Abbate C, Cutaia C, Vergani C, Bergamaschini L. Mild cognitive impairment subtypes and vascular dementia in community-dwelling elderly people: a 3-year follow-up study. *J. Am. Geriatr. Soc.* 2006 Apr;54(4):580-6.

Zaudig M. A new systematic method of measurement an diagnosis of "mild cognitive impairment" and dementia according to ICD-10 and DSM-III-R criteria. *Int. Psychogeriatr.* 1992;(Suppl 2):203-219.

Wilson RS, Barnes LL, Mendes de Leon CF, Aggarwal NT, Schneider JS, Bach J, Pilat J, Beckett LA, Arnold SE, Evans DA, Bennett DA. Depressive symptoms, cognitive decline, and risk of AD in older persons. *Neurology* 2002;59:364-370.

Wilson RS, Mendes De Leon CF, Bennett DA, Bienias JL, Evans DA. Depressive symptoms and cognitive decline in a community population of older persons. *J. Neurol. Neurosurg Psychiatry* 2004;75:126-129.

Winblad B, Palmer K, Kivipelto M, Jelic V, Fratiglioni L, Wahlund LO, Nordberg A, Backman L, Albert M, Almkvist O, Arai H, Basun H, Blennow K, de Leon M, DeCarli C, Erkinjuntti T, Giacobini E, Graff C, Hardy J, Jack C, Jorm A, Ritchie K, van Duijn C, Visser P, Petersen RC. Mild cognitive impairment--beyond controversies, towards a consensus: report of the International Working Group on Mild Cognitive Impairment. *J. Intern. Med.* 2004;256:240-246.

Wolf H, Ecke GM, Bettin S, Dietrich J, Gertz HJ. Do white matter changes contribute to the subsequent development of dementia in patients with mild cognitive impairment? A longitudinal study. *Int. J. Geriatr. Psychiatry 2000*;15:803–812.

World Health Organization. International statistical classification of diseases and related health problems, 10th revision (ICD-10). Chapter V, categories F00-F99. Mental, behavioural, and developmental disorders, *clinical description and diagnostic guidelines.* Geneva: World Health Organization, 1992

Wragg RE, Jeste DV. Overview of depression and psychosis in Alzheimer's disease. *Am. J. Psychiatry* 1989; 146: 577–589.

Yaffe K, Blackwell T, Gore R, Sands L, Reus V, Browner WS. Depressive symptoms and cognitive decline in nondemented elderly women: a prospective study. *Arch. Gen. Psychiatry* 1999;56:425-430.

In: Leading-Edge Cognitive Disorders Research
Editor: James P. Tsai, pp. 131-154

ISBN: 978-1-60021-843-9

Chapter 5

RESEARCH ON COGNITION DISORDER: METHODOLOGICAL ISSUES

Benito Pereira Damasceno[1]
Department of Neurology, Medical School,
State University of Campinas (UNICAMP),
Campinas-SP, Brazil

ABSTRACT

In this chapter we critically review and discuss methodological questions related to research on cognitive disorders. Research on this area is challenging due to the complexity of functions studied and to the numerous variables implicated. First we revisit the concept of cognition as a mediated (semiotic) and systemic activity. Accordingly, every cognitive act is carried out by a functional network of interconnected mental operations and their processing brain regions, each region belonging to various partly overlapped networks. Therefore, the result of a local lesion is not an isolated symptom but a syndrome, and the best neuropsychological approach is an analysis based on appropriate tests to disclose double dissociations and, in this way, to provide clues to brain-behavior relationships. This approach takes into account the influence of task relevant variables (confounders) related to the patient (e.g., age, education, humor state), to the lesion (size, etiology, acute versus chronic, focal versus diffuse), and to the tests and testing conditions (ecological validity, instructions, examiner´s experience, "noise"), which need to be controlled and reckoned in multivariate statistical analyses. Other controversial issues such as single and double dissociations, single-case versus group studies, and the lesion method are also examined. At the end, we illustratively bring up methodological problems of current cognitive research on early multiple sclerosis and medial temporal lobe epilepsy.

[1] E-mail: damascen@unicamp.br

Introduction

1. Cognition: Cultural-Historical and Systemic Approach

The term "cognition" (L *cognitio, cognitionis* knowledge; *cognoscere* know) is defined by Webster's Comprehensive Dictionary as "the act, power, or faculty of apprehending, knowing, or perceiving". It is a generic term that comprises functions such as attention, perception, visual-spatial-motor abilities, memory (encoding, learning, recall), language, and intellectual reasoning. Cognition has close interfunctional relationship with two other aspects of the human mind – volition and emotion, which in variable degree are constitutive of every cognitive act.

Contemporary Neuropsychology and Cognitive Neuroscience have gone beyond the old concepts of mental "faculty" and brain "center" to view the human mind as a complex activity involving interconnected mental and cerebral processes (its systemic structure), which represent the physical and social world by means of signs (its mediated, semiotic nature) and result from the internalization of external actions and relations with things and persons (its cultural-historical origin) (Vygotsky, 1934/1982; Luria, 1966/1980). This new concept of mental "function" represents a considerable theoretical-methodological contribution to basic and clinical science cognitive research.

Cognition as cultural-historical and mediated activity - The interaction of the individual with external things and phenomena is not direct or immediate, but indirect, mediated by signs (particularly the linguistic ones). From the viewpoint of an external observer, man's actions upon things seem to be direct, but these material actions are preceded by mental actions, symbolic representations, programs, and projects. In its origin, these representations or mental actions derive from the internalization of external, practical actions and relations with people and objects of the natural and cultural world. These external practices, particularly those of productive labor activity, develop under conditions of cooperation and social interaction among people, and are mediated by instruments of two kinds – material (artifacts, tools) and psychological (signs), which are social and cultural products concerning both their origin (created and improved by countless generations of human beings) and their use (learned in the joint activity with other individuals) (Vygotsky, 1978; Leontiev, 1981a, 1981b). In the appropriation of the culture by the child (cultural learning) a relevant role is played by imitation (reproduction of intentions, objectives, and cause-effect relationships perceived by the child), by children's collaborative activity with each other, and by the adult's intentional teaching (Tomasello et al., 1993). In this process of appropriation, the primary and decisive role is played by the child's practical actions with people and objects, that is, by the child's own material (object) actions, since it is a question of constructing, not the image of the action, but the ideal action, the mind as action (Galperin, 1976; Wertsch, 1998).

Cognition as a functional system - Every mental act (object perception, problem solving, discourse interpretation) is carried out by a "complex functional system" (Vygotsky, 1934/1982; Anokhin, 1935) also conceived of as "neurofunctional network" (Mesulam, 1990), "distributed parallel processing" (Rummelhart and McClelland, 1986), or "multiple drafts model" (Dennet, 1991).

This insight on mental functions was first articulated by Hughlings Jackson (1958), who conceived psychological functions as organized in different levels of complexity and abstraction (the voluntary, conscious; and the involuntary, automatic, unconscious). He also emphasized the need to distinguish between evidence for localization of *symptoms* versus the idea of localization of *function*. A starting point for Jackson's analysis of speech disturbances produced by local brain lesions was the case of a patient who, having failed to say (to repeat) the word "no", replied: "No, doctor, I never can say 'no'!". In this case, the focal lesion could impair the representation or production of the word in a level (the conscious, voluntary, decontextualized, metalinguistic), but not in the other one (involuntary, automatic).

The functional system or network comprises various basic operations (processes, mechanisms, or components) organized in a dynamic assembly of interconnected brain regions, each region giving its specific contribution to the functioning of the system as a whole. As conceived of by Gazzaniga et al. (1998), mental operations involve taking a representation as an input, performing some sort of process on the input, and then producing a new representation, or output. Thus, mental operations are processes that generate, elaborate upon, or manipulate mental representations. Consider, for example, the solving of a problem presented orally to the subject: "Anthony has 11 bananas and Mary has 6 bananas less than he has. How many bananas do they have together?". This task requires many components such as (1) the processing of the sounds in the acoustic analyzer (auditory pathways to the primary cortical area in Heschel gyri), (2) extraction and synthesis of phonemes and words in neighbouring secondary cortical areas, (3) decoding of meaning of words and sentences, as well as understanding of logical-grammatical relationships ("less than") in posterior and anterior tertiary multimodal cortical areas, (4) orientating in the data, hypothesis testing, monitoring and verifying of solution in prefrontal areas, and (5) symbolic-spatial reasoning (subtracting 11 minus 5) in inferior parietal-occipital cortex.

Every mental act has a psychological structure and cerebral organization which change from moment to moment insofar as each task or operation goes on commuting one for another. Each activity requires a different ensemble of cognitive operations suitable to achieve its objective, besides motivational and emotional components. Its objective remains constant, but the methods or basic operations can vary (Luria, 1973). This plasticity also characterizes the process of acquisition of any new ability (e.g., car driving). At first, the structure of activity is expanded and requires a number of essential aids for its performance, but afterwards it gradually becomes condensed and converted into an automatic (motor) skill. So, in the initial learning phase, the activity requires numerous mental components (conscious intention; attention; working memory; language; visual, auditory, tactile-proprioceptive, and spatial perception) and various brain regions (prefrontal, posterior parietal, premotor, basalganglia, sensory-perceptive, and so on). Later on, when skillful mastery is attained, the execution of the task becomes automatic, partly unconscious, as a kind of implicit knowledge (procedural memory) which involves fewer brain regions (premotor, motor, parietal, basalganglia circuit).

2. Neuropsychological Investigation: Methodological Issues

The objective of neuropsychological investigation is (1) to analyze the patient's symptoms by means of appropriate tests in order to diagnose an organic brain dysfunction and, by disclosing double dissociations, to establish which basic mechanism is impaired, and thus to diagnose the side and local of brain lesion; (2) to yield a baseline and profile of cognitive deficits for future comparisons, in order to evaluate the efficacy of drugs and rehabilitation programs (clinical trials), or simply to follow-up the natural history of the disease; and (3), in forensic neuropsychology, to predict the functional relationship between the patient´s performance on neuropsychological tests and his behavior in real-world settings. In this chapter we are dealing mainly with the first objective. Nowadays, the lesion local can be quickly and accurately diagnosed with computerized tomography (CT) or magnetic resonance imaging (MRI). However, conventional MRI may not show signs of lesion in a site where the neuropsychological analysis indicates there is a dysfunction, as it usually occurs in the early phase of Alzheimer´s disease, when a finding of impaired retrieval and recognition may suggest an entorhinal-hippocampal neuronal loss.

2.1. Systemic or Network Approach

At least three basic assumptions orient analysis of cognitive syndromes in Neuropsychology and Behavioral Neurology (Luria, 1966/1980; Mesulam, 1990). These assumptions are not applied to the analysis of sensory-motor symptoms such as the loss of general sensation or movement in one half of the body (hemi-hypesthesia, hemiparesis) or the loss of vision in one hemifield (hemianopsia), which indicate lesion in their respective contralateral primary cortical zones or projection pathways.

2.1.1. Each Brain Region, Particularly those in Convergence Zones, Contains the Neuralsubstratum (Basic Operation) of Different Complex Functions and Can Thus Belong to Various Partly Overlapped Neuronal Networks.

As an example, the left inferior-posterior parietal region (Brodmann´s area 39) plays relevant role in seemingly disparate tasks such as assembling the parts of a chair, reproducing a model by means of multicolored cubes, orienting to right or left in a street or in the own body, subtracting 6 from 11, and understanding logical-grammatical structures that express spatial relationships (e.g., "the father´s brother", "above", "below", "between", "before") or sentences with embedded relative clauses ("The boy *who is embraced by the brother of his father* is going to travel now"). All these different tasks require a basic operation, namely *spatial reasoning*, be it in the physical-concrete or in the abstract-symbolic level. Therefore, the neuronal networks of these tasks are partly overlapped in this brain region.

2.1.2.Lesion Limited to One Region Impairs Different Complex Mental Functions, Thus Resulting in Multiple Symptoms or Neuropsychological Syndromes.

This postulate is derived from the former. In a patient with lesion in the left inferior-posterior parietal region we usually have, not an isolated symptom, but a syndrome comprising constructive apraxia, difficulties with mental rotation of figures, acalculia, left-right desorientation, and difficulties understanding logical-grammatical constructions (Luria´s semantic aphasia).

2.1.3. Different Components of the Same Complex Function Can Be Impaired by Lesions in Different Regions or in their Interconnecting Pathways.

Each complex function (problem solving, story retelling) requires a set of different basic mental operations, particularly those processed in multimodal convergence zones such as the prefrontal (for planning, monitoring and correcting), parietal-occipital (for spatial reasoning), and entorhinal-hippocampal (for long-term explicit memorization). In case of lesions, it is not enough for the evaluating clinician to say that a complex function is impaired, by stating that the patient has an aphasia or intellectual disability. Instead he should explain in what way the complex function is impaired and establish the subtype or profile of the cognitive syndrome, which varies according to which basic component is impaired.

Syndrome analysis by means of a comprehensive battery of neuropsychological tests and appropriate control conditions can help to disclose which basic component is impaired and, by inference, which brain structure is damaged. The tests should be selected insofar as they evaluate or measure the relevant components hypothetically involved in the complex function studied. The most crucial form of control is to compare the patient´s test performance to that of healthy individuals. This is a condition for ascribing the patient´s poorer performance to his brain lesion. Sometimes, for example in studies of chronic degenerative motor neuron disease, the best control group is made up of patients with another disease (e.g., rheumatoid arthritis), similarly chronic and depressing but without lesion in the central nervous system.

Besides a control group, control tasks are needed to determine if the patient´s cognitive or behavioral problem results from dysfunction of a particular component (e.g., loss of spatial reasoning or long-term memorization) or whether it is a consequence of a more widespread disturbance (attentional deficit, depression). Consider, for example, the evaluation of memory problems of a patient with temporal lobe epilepsy. He complains forgetting names of things, messages to be delivered to another person, and local where they put their belongings (keys, eye-glasses). In this case, you suspect an impairment of declarative, episodic memory, and decide to evaluate it with appropriate tests for verbal and visual learning (word list, series of figures). The patient´s low scores on these tests can result either from a primary disturbance of episodic memory or from disorder of another component relevant to the learning tasks, such as verbal fluency, visual perception, attention, and mood state. So, you have to assess these components by means of appropriate control tests, such as WAIS-R digit span for attention (Wechsler, 1981); FAS or category (animals) for verbal fluency (Lezak, 1995); Poppelreuter´s overlapping figures (Luria, 1966/1980), Hooper visual organization (Hooper, 1983) or form discrimination test (Benton et al., 1983) for visual perception; and Beck´s scale for mood (Beck, 1987).

2.2. Single and Double Dissociations

Focal lesion of the associative cortex often affects several complex functions (e.g., constructional praxis, calculation, understanding of sentences with logical-grammatical structure), since each of these functions depends on the same basic operation (spatial reasoning) that is impaired. Nevertheless, the lesion leaves intact other functions that do not depend on this operation (e.g., speech fluency, understanding of melodies and simpler sentences, and learning of word list).

In this case, when a lesion to brain region A disrupts function X but not function Y, we have a single dissociation between the functions. The term "dissociation" refers not to the loss of association between two brain regions, but to the dissociated performance of a subject who executes extremely poorly on one task and at a normal or very much better level on another task. In a single dissociation, the difference in performance level on tasks X and Y does not mean that the two tasks require a different set of basic operations, since task X may simply be easier than task Y, which requires greater amount of cognitive resources (Shallice, 1988).

More robust conclusions about brain function can be drawn by finding another patient with the reverse condition, that is, a lesion to region B, which disrupts function Y while leaving function X intact. Then, we can establish a double dissociation, a concept introduced by Teuber (1955), and further developed by Weiskrantz (1968), Kinsbourne (1971), and Shallice (1988). With this concept we can make more specific inferences about brain function even in functional neuroimaging studies of normal subjects. For example, consider two brain regions, A and B, and two experimental tasks, X and Y: during execution of task X, region A is active, but B is not, the converse occurring during performance of task Y. Since one experimental manipulation has an effect on A but not on B and another on B but not on A, the conclusion can be drawn that these regions have different functional properties (Huettel et al., 2004).

2.3. Single-Case Versus Group Studies

The experimental method consists in isolating and testing individual variables in order to verify possible cause-effect relationships or, at least, associations between events. In this regard, a case-control design is commonly adopted. To satisfy the homogeneity principle, all cases should have the same kind of lesion (e.g., infarction), and all cases and controls should be identical in all influential variables except in that which is being studied. The problem is that brain lesions produced by natural diseases (stroke, multiple sclerosis, Alzheimer´s disease) are never exactly alike, they vary from patient to patient as regards their size, distribution, and mental-behavioral manifestations. This anatomical and behavioral variability between patients indicates that different functional subsystems are damaged, and creates difficulties when including these patients into a single lesion group (e.g., parietal or frontal). Furthermore, group studies may present practical difficulties. Due to the strict selection criteria, it may take a long time to collect enough patients, and even when the patients fulfill these criteria, they may not be in condition of being tested or willing to be so at the appropriate time (Shallice, 1988).

Due to these limitations of group studies, some authors (Caramazza, 1992) have argued that single case studies can contribute to better understanding of cognitive processes, by comprehensively analyzing the performance of individual patients and making comparisons across multiple cases. Damasio and Damasio (1989) also consider as the ideal approach the collection of and reflection on multiple single-case studies, particularly those based on high level sophistication of cognitive construct and anatomical-neuroimaging resolution. In fact, the detailed study of individual cases can yield more information than great series (groups) in which many potentially interesting findings would not be reckoned in the statistical handling of the data. According to Gazzaniga et al., (2002), the single case study method affords powerful insights into the functional components of cognition, as exemplified by Caramazza´s study of patients with category-specific anomia. One of these patients showed a consistent and striking disability in naming fruits and vegetables, but no impairment in naming objects such as tools or furniture (Hart et al., 1985), thus supporting a category-specific organization of the mental lexicon.

The problem with single case studies is their limitation for linking cognitive operations to neural structures, even in patients with unique cognitive deficits associated to a focal cortical lesion (Gazzaniga et al. 2002). It is difficult to know which affected region is correlated to the deficit, since the lesion usually involves several disparate cortical structures plus the underlying white matter, besides every patient having idiosyncrasies in their cognitive-cerebral organization, so that a lesion of same local, size and nature in different subjects can produce different syndromes. Even more controversial is the viewpoint of some cognitive psychologists who take into account exclusively what happens in the cognitive system, without regard to the underlying cerebral processes. Their inferences are based only on data collected from isolated single cases, without comparison to data extracted from suitable control subjects, and their theoretical constructs may have nothing to do with true psychological functions or, even less, with physiological cerebral functions (Crick, 1989). Comparison of patient´s performance to that of control or normative group is needed to avoid Type I errors. In many single-case studies, the sample size of the control or normative group is typically small (5 to 10 subjects), and Crawford and Garthwaite (2006) suggest an increase in control sample size to 20-30 in future single-case studies to achieve a marked effect on power and reduction of Type I errors.

Group studies can yield better insights into brain-behavior correlations. A method frequently used to establish the effective lesion site is by including in a group all patients with a particular deficit, superimposing the positions of their lesions, and looking for a "hot spot", where all lesions overlap (Shallice, 1988). The use of this method can be illustrated by Dronkers´ study of patients with apraxia of speech (Dronkers, 1996; Dronkers et al., 2000). In this study, all 25 patients had a single cerebral infarction evaluated at least one year after the stroke, and they were native English-speaking, right-handed, with normal vision and hearing and no previous neurological or psychiatric disease. Their lesions were reconstructed onto templates and superimposed by means of a microcomputer running software. Lesion overlapping showed that all patients had involvement of a discrete area of the superior tip of the precentral gyrus of the insula. As control to avoid possible artifacts, the authors evaluated 19 patients with nearly as large lesions within the left cerebral hemisphere, but without apraxia of speech, and their lesions spared the part of precentral gyrus that was damaged in all patients with this disorder (see figure 1).

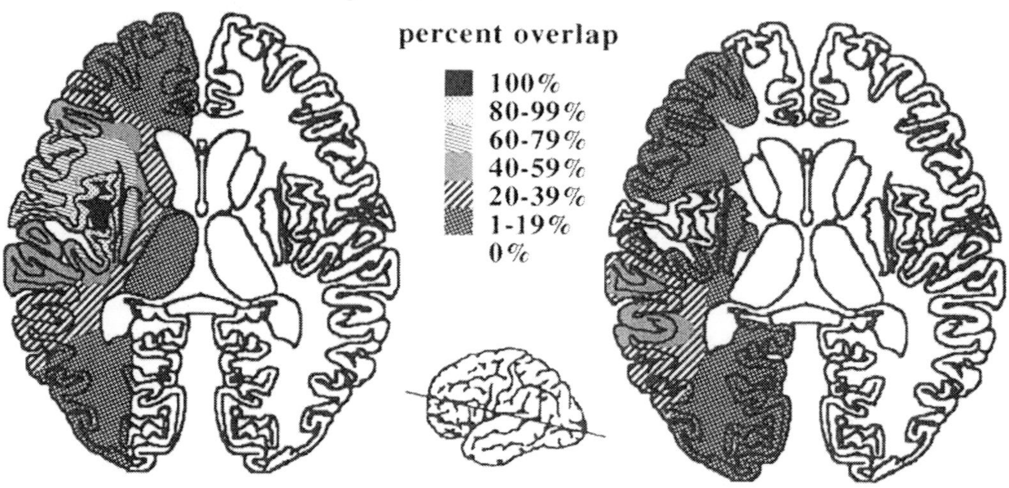

Figure 1. Lesion overlapping in 25 patients with apraxia of speech (left) and 19 patients without this disorder (right). All of the 25 patients with apraxia of speech have a lesion encompassing a small section of the insula, as shown in black, while the lesions of the 19 patients without apraxia of speech completely spare the same area. (From Dronkers et al., 2000. In: M. S. Gazzaniga editor, The new cognitive neurosciences, The MIT Press, with permission.).

2.4. Influential Variables to be Controlled

Neuropsychological assessment and particularly the interpretation of its findings is a challenging task, due to the complexity of functions evaluated and to the great number of variables involved. These variables concern the patient, its brain lesion, the tests employed, and testing conditions.

2.4.1. Patient Variables

Every patient has peculiar characteristics, which influence test performance. Particularly age and education should always be considered when matching control subjects for cognitive studies. Cognitive abilities depend on *age* and they may not be fully developed in children and adolescents, or have suffered some deterioration in normal aging. Part of age effect is due to cultural differences. Our cognitive-cerebral organization also depends on *educational and cultural experience*. Individuals with illiteracy or low educational level have difficulties with metalinguistic tests, especially those requiring pen and paper. They have difficulties to understand test instructions, and show an attitude of suspicion or aversion towards the tests. *Handedness* should also be taken into account when comparing lesion groups. There can be left hemisphere dominance for language in right-handed and variable linguistic-cognitive hemisphere dominance in ambidextrous and left-handed subjects. As regards *sex*, the most consistent finding has been a better performance of women in verbal fluency and of men in visual-spatial reasoning tasks. *Polyglotism* may also influence cognition, since certain peculiarities of every idiom (e.g., right-left versus left-right or up-down handwriting, phonologic versus ideographic type) have their specific cognitive-cerebral processing mechanisms. These differences lead to variations of syndromes in each idiom mastered by the same subject. *Personality*, *autobiography*, *affective and behavioral patterns*, *previous experience with the proposed test* or similar cognitive tasks such as checkers or chess playing, puzzle solving and hunting can influence test performance and reaction to brain lesion. Personality changes may constitute the fundamental core of the resultant neuropsychological syndrome. Other influential variables are *motivation*, *interest*, *anxiety*, *restlessness*, *depression*, and *side effect of drugs*. An often neglected variable is the *circadian variation of cognitive functions*, whose performance is worse between 12 a.m. and 2 p.m. and after 23 hours.

2.4.2. Lesion Characteristics

Neuropsychological syndromes vary according with local (brain region, focal versus multifocal or diffuse), size, nature (etiology), speed of installation, and age of lesion. With reference to speed of installation, for instance, multifocal and diffuse brain lesions can produce either a confusional state (delirium) or dementia, depending on their rapid (acute) or slow (chronic) course, respectively. Comparative studies should include patient groups of same lesion age, since the clinical syndrome changes as the time passes ("syndromenwandel"; Leischner, 1972), as typically happens with global a aphasia evolving to a Broca´s aphasia.

2.4.3. Tests

Task performance is influenced by the kind of stimulus employed (visual, tactile, or acoustic-verbal), its intensitiy and complexity. Also relevant are the presence (or not) of previous instructions, the ecological validity of the test, and its metacognitive or artificial character. Tests ecologically adapted, with tasks similar to those of every day life, are easier to be executed.

2.4.4. Testing Conditions

Other equally important variables to be controlled for are the examiner´s experience with the test, the patient´s acquaintance with the examiner, and the presence of incommodious light, temperature, or noise in the local of testing. Other "noises" to be avoided are everything that distracts the attention of the patient, for instance, a framed picture of fighting pirates on the wall, the examiner´s improper dress or ill-humored look, and the examination table with too many things in disarray. This quiet testing environment as well as the control of most influential variables are crucial for establishing brain-behavior relationships, as recommended by Lezak (1995). However, this "sterile environment" and the tests employed may be inadequate when the objective of neuropsychological evaluation is to predict (generalize) the patient´s behavior in noisy real-world settings, at home, workplace or community, hence the need to develop ecologically valid tests and testing situations (Sbordone and Long, 1996).

2.5. Brain-Behavioral Correlations: The Lesion Method

Brain lesion as result of natural disease, surgical resection or experimental ablation in animals is usually accompanied by functional disturbances in other interconnected and seemingly intact regions, due to immediate changes in neurotransmission, excitation-inhibition balance, and blood flow (dyaschisis phenomenon of von Monakow, 1910), besides mass effect, changes in cerebrospinal fluid dynamics, secondary axonal degeneration, and sometimes septic complications and non-intentional damage to neighbouring structures. Other brain regions normally activated or inhibited by the injured one are denervated and may become hypo- or hyperactive. Disturbance of excitation-inhibition balance plus functional reorganization in other brain regions play some role in the resultant syndrome, which should not be interpreted as merely the product of a subtractive maneuver, that is, by loss of the function supposedly performed by the damaged area (Fuster, 1989). Thus, to localize a lesion by neuroimaging does not imply to localize in the same region the symptoms (syndrome) or the impaired or lost function. Furthermore, natural lesions are often not well demarcated or limited to a precise neuroanatomical structure whose specific functional role one would like to investigate. In spite of these limitations, the lesion method based on clinical-anatomical correlations has been the one that most contributed to our knowledge of the cerebral organization of psychological processes, particularly before the imaging era.

Damasio and Damasio (1989, 1997) point the following prerequisites for a valid brain-behavioral correlation: (1) to choose appropriate neuropathological specimens and adequate timing for neuroimaging and concomitant neuropsychological testing; (2) to gather sufficient images for anatomical diagnosis; and (3) to interpret the group data, taking into account individual variations in neural-cognitive organization, age, sex, education, as well as psychological and social characteristics of the subjects. According to these authors, the most suitable lesions for behavioral and anatomical studies are: (a) strokes, particularly nonhemorrhagic infarction in chronic stage (more than three months old); followed by (b) resolved herpes simplex virus encephalitis, and (c) neurosurgical ablation of tumor or of epileptic focus. In cerebral infarctions, particularly in the chronic phase, the abnormal signal area seen on CT or MRI corresponds to actual destruction of brain parenchyma, while in space-occupying lesions as hemorrhage and infiltrating tumors, much of the abnormal area does contain functionally competent neurons.

The problem with surgical removal of epileptic focus is that some patients may have widespread brain abnormalities due to long-standing seizure discharges, particularly in those with multifocal or bilateral epileptogenic activity. Other epileptic patients may have disorders of neuronal migration (e.g., micropolygyria), which are sometimes unseen on conventional MRI, requiring curvilinear reconstruction technique to be detected. The inclusion of such patients in lesion studies must be evaluated on an individual basis, giving preference to those which had a consistently unilateral epileptogenic focus prior to the surgery, and are in seizure-free state after a well delimited surgical resection (e.g., medial temporal lobe removal or amygdalohippocampectomy for treatment of medial temporal lobe epilepsy).

2.6. Cognitive Research on Early Multiple Sclerosis

Multiple sclerosis (MS) is a chronic inflammatory, demyelinating disease of the central white matter, characterized by lesions (plaques) disseminated in space and time, with predilection for the optic nerve, periventricular region, and cervical cord. Sensory-motor symptoms are the most common initial manifestations of MS, presenting as a clinically isolated syndrome (CIS), which is usually related to lesion in the optic nerve, spinal cord, brain stem, or cerebellum. Rarely the first manifestation (attack) is cognitive-behavioral, with epileptic seizures, confusional psychosis, aphasia, apraxia, agnosia, memory deficits, or dementia (Achiron et al., 1992; Okuda et al., 1996; Pelosi et al., 1997). There seems to be no specific pattern of cognitive deterioration in MS, and the picture of "subcortical dementia" occurs only in 12% of patients (Beatty, 1992; Amato et al., 2001).

In hospital-based studies, most of them cross-sectional, estimates of the prevalence of cognitive dysfunction in MS vary widely, with reported rates ranging between 13 and 65% (Peyser et al., 1990; Rao, 1997). This wide variation in prevalence is influenced by the method used for evaluation of cognitive function, and by the heterogeneity of cases studied as regards their clinical course, degree of disability, disease duration, localization and number of lesions, and severity of cognitive deficits. Probably, cognitive dysfunction in the general MS population is not so high, since 20% of patients with MS have a benign form of the disease (McAlpine, 1964).

In the few longitudinal investigations hitherto undertaken, cognitive disturbances often appear early in the course of the disease, even in the clinically isolated syndrome (CIS), when MS diagnosis is only "probable" or "possible" (Rao et al., 1991; Amato et al., 2001; Achiron and Barak, 2000; Achiron and Barak, 2003). First and most affected have been verbal memory, abstract reasoning and linguistic processes, followed by impairment of sustained attention and short-term spatial memory; and these cognitive deficits have a highly negative impact on work and social activities, independent of degree of physical disability (Grant et al., 1984; Amato et al., 2001). Cognitive impairment is related to axonal loss and brain atrophy, which occur early in the course of the disease (De Stefano et al., 2001; Deloire et al., 2005). Degree of cognitive impairment and physical disability level are independent predictors of handicap in the workplace and in social settings, as shown by Amato et al. (2001) in a 10 years follow-up study of 45 MS patients.

In most MS patients, the disease presents as a progressive cognitively disabling process, which needs to be diagnosed as early as possible for the treatment to be more effective, since various multicenter clinical trials with disease modifying medications (beta-interferon) have shown beneficial effects on the rate of conversion of CIS to clinically definite MS and on improving cognitive functions (Jacobs et al., 2000; Comi et al., 2001; Kappos et al., 2006). In this regard, McDonald et al. (2001) criteria have represented a significant step for the early diagnosis of MS, by taking into account MRI findings of dissemination in time and space, even in the absence of any new clinical symptom of the disease. According to these criteria, an "attack" (relapse) is defined as "an episode of neurological disturbance of the kind seen in MS, lasting for at least 24 hours, when clinicopathological studies have established that the causative lesions are inflammatory and demyelinating in nature". The problem is that most neurologists consider as "attack" only sensory-motor manifestations of the disease, such as paresis, sensory loss, paresthesia, ataxia, optic neuritis, and transverse myelitis. Initial cognitive-behavioral disturbance is usually considered as atypical for MS and undervalued for the diagnosis and prognosis of the disease, unless a MS-typical second attack or new MRI lesion takes place.

Another problem for the study of cognition in early MS, as Achiron and Barak (2006) called attention to, is that there is no consensus in the neurological literature regarding (1) the definition of the temporal phase of the disease course termed "early"; (2) what constitutes cognitive impairment; and (3) what tools are necessary to assess cognition in early MS.

In order to establish the diagnosis as soon as possible, MS "early phase" could be defined, according to Achiron and Barak (2006), as (a) immediately at the onset of new neurological symptoms of predominantly white matter involvement suggestive of MS; or (b) within the time till the occurrence of a second neurological event. "Cognitive impairment" is defined by most authors with the "all or none" approach, based on existence or absence of any cognitive abnormality (Achiron et al., 2005); or the "categorical" approach, by classifying the number of failed cognitive subtests into sets, which represent the extent of cognitive decline, as did Amato et al. (2001) (0 to 2 tests failed, no impairment; 3 to 5, mild impairment; and >5, moderate impairment).

As yet there is no consensus among clinicians regarding the best tools to assess cognition in early MS. Most MS clinics and neurological practices do not routinely assess cognition. In clinical trials, the disease is usually evaluated by means of the Expanded Disability Status Scale (EDSS; Kurtzke, 1983), which is biased towards the sensory-motor function, and presents problems with standardization and poor inter-rater reliability. The introduction of the MS Functional Composite (MSFC; Cutter et al., 1999) has offered several advantages insofar as it is standardized, reproducible, more sensitive to change in neurological status, and has a cognitive test (the paced auditory serial addition test, PASAT), besides the testing of arm and hand function (the nine-hole peg test), leg function and ambulation (a 25-foot timed walk). However, MSFC assessment of cognition with PASAT (in which the subject has to add each number to the one immediately preceding it while numbers are presented orally every three seconds) is limited to attention and working memory.

Several screening tests have been used in MS, such as the Mini-Mental State Examination (MMSE; Folstein et al., 1975), the Clock Drawing Test (CDT; Barak et al., 2002), and the MS Neuropsychological Screening Questionnaire (MSNQ; Benedict et al., 2003). These tests have limited power to diagnose cognitive impairment, particularly the MMSE, whose sensitivity ranges from 28 to 36%, and specificity from 89 to 100% (Swirsky-Sacchetti et al., 1992). Another limitation of MMSE in MS patients is that it requires good hand and visual functions, which are frequently compromised by paresis, ataxia, or optic neuritis. Alternative screening tests more suitable for MS patients with such physical disabilities are the Short Orientation-Memory-Concentration test (SOMC; Katzman et al., 1983) and the Cognitive Abilities Screening Instrument – Short version (CASI-S; Teng et al., 1998; Damasceno et al., 2005), which contain the most predictive items found in MMSE, namely register, recall, and orientation (Magaziner et al., 1987).

In order to avoid the limitations of screening tests, brief neuropsychological batteries have been developed, which cover the functions most often compromised in MS. The most widely used are the Brief Repeatable Battery of Neuropsychological tests (BRB-N; Boringa et al., 2001) and the Neuropsychological Screening Battery for Multiple Sclerosis (NSBMS; Rao et al., 1991). The BRB-N comprises the following tests: (1) the selective reminding test (SRT) for verbal learning of a list of 12 words presented in five consecutive trials, followed by its recall after an 11 minute delay; (2) the 10/36 spatial recall test (SPART) for visual learning and delayed recall by reproducing the pattern of 10 checkers on a 6x6 checkerboard viewed for 10 seconds; (3) the symbol digit modalities test (SDMT) for selective attention and concentration by associating symbols with numbers during 90 seconds; (4) the paced auditory serial addition test (PASAT) for information processing speed, sustained attention and working memory; and (5) the word list generation (WLG) for semantic verbal fluency by spontaneously producing words beginning with a particular letter during 60 seconds. BRB-N is a sensitive measure of cognitive impairment in early MS, but it is influenced by age, education, and physical disability, besides showing significant practice effect in the PASAT subtest (Bever et al., 1995). PASAT scores can also be influenced by dysarthria, in spite of normal cognitive function.

Thus, it is challenging to study complex mental functions in a disease which is also complex, even in its early phase, in which neuropsychological evaluation can disclose cognitive impairment, whose prevalence has varied from 26% (Amato et al., 2001) to 53.7% (Achiron and Barak, 2003). In this phase of the disease, MR spectroscopy and magnetization transfer imaging have shown signs of widespread axonal degeneration in the normal appearing white matter (outside the plaques) (Rovaris et al., 1998; Rovaris et al., 2006), which is correlated to cognitive deterioration, fatigue, and depression. Most recent studies have used comprehensive neuropsychological batteries to test the cognitive functions often affected in MS, but without employing control tasks (counterproofs) to verify the influence of confounding variables on the tests proposed; or without analyzing this possible influence by means of appropriate statistical tests. In Amato´s et al. study (2001), for instance, 22 (44%) of 50 MS patients had depression as classified by the Hamilton Rating Scale, but the influence of this variable on cognitive performance was not statistically analyzed. Another limitation of most studies is that the evaluation of episodic memory (e.g., word list learning and delayed recall) is restricted to the processes of encoding and free recall, leaving recognition untested, and for this reason being incapable to conclude about the memory mechanism affected. Low scores on free delayed recall of word list may be explained by encoding or retrieval deficiency, which may be related to anxiety, depression, fatigue, drug effect, or to any kind of executive dysfunction, unless a poor recognition performance discloses that the consolidation process is faulty, thus suggesting an entorhinal-hippocampal dysfunction.

2.7. Medial Temporal Lobe Epilepsy

Temporal lobe epilepsy is the most common partial epilepsy in adults, often associated with mesial temporal sclerosis, memory decline, and drug resistance, but presenting good postoperative outcome. The seizures usually arise from the medial temporal region (amygdala, hippocampus, parahippocampal gyrus) characterizing the so called medial temporal lobe epilepsy (MTLE), which may present as a simple (SPS) or complex partial seizure (CPS). SPS may occur isolated or immediately preceding a CPS. Common symptoms in SPS are a rising epigastric sensation, fear, "déjà vu" or "jamais vu" experience, sudoresis, paleness, and occasionally olfactory and gustative sensations. CPS is characterized by motor stop, stare, pupil dilation and oromandibular and/or manual automatisms, with duration ranging from 1 to 2 minutes. In the post-ictal period, the patient may exhibit mental confusion, disorientation, and impairment of memory and language. CPS may further evolve to a secondarily generalized tonic-clonic seizure. The presence of auditory illusion or hallucination, dizziness, or sudden speech arrest in the beginning of the seizure suggests involvement of lateral temporal cortex.

In the interictal period, these patients may present difficulties with memory, concentration, and reasoning, as well as astheno-emotional, depressive, and rarely psychotic disturbances. These cognitive-behavioral problems may be related to the epilepsy itself, to the underlying brain lesion, to side effect of antiepileptic drugs (AED), or to a combination of these factors. AEDs, particularly phenobarbital, primidon, and phenytoin, may cause cognitive disorders similar to those of epilepsy itself, even when their serum concentration is in the therapeutic range.

In the investigation, electroencephalography (EEG) may be normal or show non-epileptiform (slow waves) and/or epileptiform discharges (acute waves), unilateral or bilateral, synchronous or asynchronous, in the anterior temporal regions. Interictal single photon emission computed tomography (SPECT) may show areas of hypoperfusion in temporal region, whereas ictal SPECT may delimit areas of hyperperfusion in the same region, corresponding to the epileptogenic focus (Engel et al., 1997). Magnetic resonance imaging (MRI) may be normal or show decrease of hippocampal volume in T1 acquisitions and increase of signal in T2 acquisitions, which are correlated to characteristic pathologic changes of hippocampal sclerosis (Engel et al., 1997; Cendes et al., 1993a; Cendes et al., 1993b; Cendes and Kobayashi, 2000). The volume reduction may further extend to other structures of the mesial temporal region, and even to the entire lateral temporal lobe, unilateral or bilaterally, often asymmetric (Cendes and Kobayashi, 2000). Pathologically, chronic MTLE is accompanied by progressive neuronal loss and astrocytic proliferation (mesial temporal sclerosis, MTS) in the amygdala, hippocampal fields CA1, CA3 and CA4 (with relative preservation of CA2), dentate gyrus, and parahippocampal gyrus (Heinemann et al., 1996). MTLE is related to familial history of epilepsy, febrile seizures in infancy, and previous status epilepticus (Engel et al., 1997; Cendes et al., 1993a).

Neuropsychological evaluation is generally normal, except for a mild-to-moderate memory deficit observed in most patients with not well-controlled seizures (Engel et al., 1997). This memory impairment affects the conscious learning of new material (verbal or non-verbal), and is correlated to the hippocampal atrophy detected by RM volumetry and cell counting of this region (Jones-Gotman et al., 1993; Sass et al., 1991). Studies of MTLE patients have shown a material-specific deficit of memory, with lesions of left hippocampus affecting verbal memory, and those of right hippocampus, visual memory (Milner, 1958; Hermann et al., 1995; Jones-Gotman, 1996). Nevertheless, more recent studies have shown that the relationship between side of hippocampal pathology and memory dysfunction is more evident in left than in right MTLE (Hermann et al., 1997; Wilde et al., 2001; Leone et al., 2001; Alessio et al., 2004). Moreover, this material-specific memory model was constructed on the basis of temporal lobectomy case studies. Few studies have tested its validity in unoperated patients (Jones-Gotman et al., 1997; Baxendale et al., 1998; Gleissner et al., 2002).

Medial temporal lobe and memory - Functional differences (double dissociations) have been found between side (left versus right) and subregions of the medial temporal lobe (MTL). The amygdala is involved in implicit, emotional memory, while the hippocampus and neighbouring cortical structures play a critical role in the formation of explicit memories.

Selective and bilateral lesions of the amygdala prevent fear conditioning in humans without impairing explicit memory for the events that occurred during the experimental testing, while similar lesions in the hippocampus interfere with acquisition of episodic memory, but not with fear conditioning (Bechara et al., 1995). In experiments using PET-scan or MRI, long term memory for emotionally charged stimuli correlates to amygdala activation, which predominates at the right side when frightening vocal expressions or unpleasant words are used as stimuli (Hamann et al., 1999; Phillips et al., 1998; Kiehl et al., 1998; Tabert et al., 2001).

The hippocampus, on the other hand, plays relevant role in explicit long term learning, particularly when a spatial component is present in the task situation. It has been shown that the hippocampus stores a cognitive map of the spatial layout of an environment (O´Keefe and Nadel, 1978). The right hippocampus and parahippocampal cortex are crucial for learning the spatial location of objects (Bohbot et al., 1998; Smith and Milner, 1981), especially when the position of each object is registered automatically and unintentionally. The parahippocampal cortex seems to be engaged in the intersection of perception and memory, and it mediates the extended persistence of cortical representations of memory. Animal studies have shown that the parahippocampal cortex is particularly important for recognition memory, and that selective lesions to this region severely impair memory (Suzuki et al., 1993). However, the role of the parahippocampal regions in the memory deficits exhibited by MTLE patients is not yet completely understood. In our study using MRI volumetry of MTL subregions in these patients (Alessio et al., 2006), we could not find correlation between this region and memory as measured by Wechsler Memory Scale, probably because this test battery is not robust enough to detect such a correlation.

Preoperative neuropsychological evaluation of memory in MTLE - The main challenge is to establish the side and site of the temporal lobe dysfunction based on results of neuropsychological testing alone, without knowing the clinical-electroencephalographic and MRI and/or SPECT data. When the data from these three sources point to the same side and local of brain dysfunction (epileptic focus and/or MTS), then we can make a safer surgical decision and predict good postoperative outcome, with long-term reduction or elimination of seizures in 58% to 64% of the cases (Wiebe et al., 2001; Tellez-Zenteno et al., 2006). The best surgical results are achieved when all EEGs (particularly with video-EEG and ictal SPECT) register a consistently unilateral epileptogenic focus, whose side is the same of MTS seen on MRI and of memory deficit disclosed by neuropsychological testing.

The endeavor of epilepsy surgery is to remove the epileptogenic focus completely without significant side effects, but this procedure may sometimes results in memory decline. As a rule, the larger the degree of preoperative hippocampal atrophy and memory deficit, the smaller the risk of postoperative worsening of this cognitive function (Baxendale et al., 1997; Loring and Meador, 1997). Conversely, resection of an epileptogenic hippocampus that is structurally intact and presents good memory function may lead to a more evident amnesia (Trenerry et al., 1993).

Neuropsychological evaluation should comprise cognition, emotion, personality, and quality of life, which use to deteriorate in the chronic course of epilepsy. First step is not the cognitive testing itself, but an initial interview with the patient, which contribute to establish empathy and to avoid future "noise" in the testing, as well as to get some idea on his intellectual level, worries, attitudes, personality, and premorbid skills. Knowledge of premorbid skills is relevant for interpretation of a patient´s test scores. For example, an average score on a test of mental arithmetic would represent a marked decline from the premorbid level in a patient who was a qualified accountant, while a score below the normative mean does not necessarily represent an acquired deficit in an individual who had modest premorbid abilities (Crawford and Garthwaite, 2002). Following the interview comes the application of a basic test battery, which in most epilepsy center includes an estimate of pre-morbid cognitive competence and intelligence with the Wechsler Adult Intelligence Scale – Revised; assessment of attention with WAIS-R digit span; visual-spatial perception with Rey Complex Figure; Osterrieth, 1944), language (Boston Naming, FAS Verbal Fluency, Token Test) (Kaplan et al., 1983; Lezak, 1995; De Renzi and Vignolo, 1962), memory (Wechsler Memory Scale – Revised or Rey Auditory Verbal Learning) (Wechsler, 1987; Rey, 1964), and mental flexibility (Stroop, Wisconsin Card Sorting, Trail Making) (Stroop, 1935; Heaton et al., 1993; Lezak, 1995).

Memory assessment is the most important component of the whole cognitive testing in patients with MTLE, due to the relevant role of MTL structures in memory functioning and to the high prevalence of memory impairment in these patients. As emphasized by Milner (1971) and Jones-Gotman (1996), memory testing should take into account the functional difference between the two temporal lobes: the left (dominant) temporal lobe mediates memory for verbal material, such as names, word lists or number sequences, and the right temporal lobe mediates memory for material that cannot be readily verbalized, such as faces, places, or abstract designs. Thus, in order to detect a double dissociation in the functions of both temporal lobes, (1) the test material should be highly polarized as for its verbal versus non-verbal character (for example, list of abstract words versus abstract designs); (2) the tests ought to be learning tasks, with repeated presentation of the material, so unimpaired individuals can improve with additional exposure to the material, increasing the difference between people with a true learning deficit and those who do poorly on a first trial for other reasons; and (3) the tests should be matched as regards the kind of memory activity they require (recall or recognition), varying only according to the verbal versus non-verbal nature of the material (Jones-Gotman,1996). According to this author, two of the most used tests (Wechsler Memory Scale and Rey Complex Figure) are not well polarized into the verbal versus non-verbal nature of their material nor are they matched as concerns the kind of memory activity involved, so they are not fit for comparisons between the hemispheres.

Neuropsychological and MRI data may not be sufficient to determine the risk of language or memory impairment following mesial temporal lobectomies, especially when the investigation show signs of bitemporal dysfunction, for instance, bilateral EEG or MRI changes, presence of epileptogenic focus in one side and hippocampal atrophy in the other, and deficit of both verbal and visual memory. In these cases, the additional contribution of the intracarotid Amytal test (IAT) is decisive. IAT procedure consists in injecting 150 to 175 mg sodium amobarbital into the internal carotid artery (via femoral catheter) to inactivate the ipsilateral hemisphere in order to test language and memory functions of the unanesthetized contralateral hemisphere. Although considered the gold standard, the IAT has a series of limitations: (1) it is an invasive procedure; (2) it has poor spatial resolution, since almost the entire hemisphere is anesthetized during the test, including the anterior and medial regions of entorhinal and hippocampal cortices; (3) each cerebral hemisphere is tested separately; (4) it is susceptible to errors that may arise due to excessive and inadequate anesthesia, or abnormal vasculature; (5) it offers a too narrow time window for detailed cognitive testing; (7) it has limited ability to distinguish verbal versus visual memory deficits; (8) in spite of its predictive value, it may show false-positives, since there are case reports of inconsistent results in repeated procedures and of positive results in patients that did not exhibit amnesia following surgery (Aldenkamp et al., 2003; Novelly and Williamson, 1989).

These limitations of IAT have led some researchers to explore alternative methods, especially functional magnetic resonance imaging (fMRI) (Golby et al., 2002). In fMRI experiments, cerebral regions are activated by stimuli or tasks presented in blocked or event-related design, with subsequent vasodilation of arterioles, capillaries and venules, increase in blood flow and in the ratio of oxygenated to deoxygenated hemoglobin, creating the BOLD (blood-oxygenation-level dependent) contrast, which is the basis for image construction. This is not a straightforward image of the brain, but a statistical map overlaid on a normalized anatomical MRI image, whose colors indicate the probability that the findings could occur under the null hypothesis. fMRI has some advantages over IAT: (1) it is a non-invasive imaging technique; (2) it activates brain regions while IAT is an inactivation procedure; (3) it has high spatial resolution; (4) the cerebral hemispheres are tested simultaneously; (5) it yields sufficient time for detailed evaluation of language and memory functions; (6) it allows sequential studies for a better characterization of the pre- and postoperative memory deficits. In fact, fMRI can show activation of areas crucial to task performance, but usually there are other wider spread activations difficult to be interpreted. fMRI has limitations that should be taken into account when drawing conclusions about brain function on the basis of its results (Jezzard et al., 2001; Huettel et al., 2004): (1) it has limited time resolution, since cortical neuronal responses occur within tens of milliseconds following a stimulus, while the first observable hemodynamic changes do not occur until 1 to 2 seconds later; (2) it may present artifacts related particularly to magnetic susceptibility changes in the frontal and temporal lobes, which use to be areas of interest in fMRI studies of MTLE patients; and these artifacts tend to increase the higher the magnetic field of the MRI equipment.

In summary, memory disturbance in MTLE is the result of interplay of the epileptic focus, the underlying brain lesion (MTS), and side effect of AEDs. Other influential variables are an earlier age at seizure onset, longer duration of epilepsy, and higher seizure frequency. MTS in its turn is associated with a family history of epilepsy, febrile seizures in infancy, and previous status epilepticus. The interplay is even more complex if we consider memory as part of a network where it has interfunctional relationships with other psychological variables, such as mood state, attention, perception, executive function, and IQ. These variables can affect performance on memory tasks and need to be controlled and considered in a multiple regression (as backward stepwise regression) or multivariate statistical analysis (as ANCOVA), otherwise the finding of low memory scores cannot be explained by a memory specific impairment.

CONCLUSION

Contemporary Neuropsychology and Cognitive Neuroscience have gone beyond the old concepts of mental "faculty" and brain "center" to view the human mind as a complex activity mediated by signs and involving various interconnected mental and cerebral processes. Research on cognition disorder has to take into account this network structure of cognitive functions (be it attention, memory, language, or intellect) and their relationships with each other and with volition and emotion. Methodologically, particularly in a brain-behavior correlation study, the researcher has to consider the influence of task relevant variables by means of suitable control conditions in order to disclose double dissociations, which may suggest what basic mental component is impaired and, by inference, what brain region is damaged. In this kind of study, it is crucial to choose appropriate neuropathological specimens and adequate timing for neuroimaging and concomitant neuropsychological testing, and to interpret the group data taking into account individual variations in neural-cognitive organization, age, sex, education, as well as psychological and social-cultural characteristics of the subjects. Both methods – qualitative and quantitative, single-case and group studies are valid, depending on the objective of the research.

REFERENCES

Achiron, A; Barak, Y. Multiple sclerosis - from probable to definite diagnosis: a 7-year prospective study. *Archives of Neurology*, 2000, 57, 974-979.

Achiron, A; Barak, Y. Cognitive impairment in probable multiple sclerosis. *Journal of Neurology, Neurosurgery, and Psychiatry*, 2003, 74, 443-446.

Achiron, A; Barak, Y. Cognitive changes in early MS: a call for a common framework. *Journal of the Neurological Sciences*, 2006, 245, 47-51.

Achiron, A; Ziv, I; Djaldetti, R; Goldberg, H; Kuritzky, A; Melamed, E. Aphasia in multiple sclerosis: clinical and radiological correlations. *Neurology*, 1992, 42, 2195-2197.

Achiron, A; Polliack, M; Rao, SM; Barak, Y; Lavie, M; Appelboim, N; Harel, Y. Cognitive patterns and progression in multiple sclerosis: construction and validation of percentile curves. *Journal of Neurology, Neurosurgery, and Psychiatry*, 2005, 76, 744-749.

Aldenkamp, AP; Boon, PA; Deblaere, K; Achten, E; Backes, WH; Boon, P; Hofman, P; Troost, J; Vandemaele, P; Vermeulen, J; Vonck, K; Wilmink, J. Usefulness of language and memory testing during intracarotid amobarbital testing: observations from an fMRI study. *Acta Neurologica Scandinavica*, 2003, 108, 147-152.

Alessio, A; Damasceno, BP; Camargo, HP; Kobayashi, E; Guerreiro, CAM; Cendes, F. Differences in memory performance and other clinical characteristics in patients with mesial temporal lobe epilepsy with and without hippocampal atrophy. *Epilepsy and Behavior*, 2004, 5, 22-27.

Alessio, A; Bonilha, L; Damasceno, BP; Kobayashi, E; Min, LL; Cendes, F. Memory and language impairments and their relationships to hippocampal and perirhinal cortex damage in patients with medial temporal lobe epilepsy. *Epilepsy and Behavior* 2006, 8, 593-600.

Amato, MP; Ponziani, G; Siracusa, G; Sorbi, S. Cognitive dysfunction in early-onset multiple sclerosis: a reappraisal after 10 years. *Archives of Neurology*, 2001, 58, 1602-1606.

Anokhin, PK. Problems of center and periphery in the physiology of nervous activity. Gorki: Gozizdat; 1935. (in Russian)

Barak, Y; Lavie, M; Achiron, A. Screening for early cognitive impairment in multiple sclerosis patients using the clock drawing test. *Journal of Clinical Neuroscience*, 2002, 9, 629-632.

Baxendale, SA; van Paesschen, W; Thompson, PJ; Duncan, JS; Shorvon, SD; Connelly, A. The relation between quantitative MRI measures of hippocampal structure and the intracarotid amobarbital test. *Epilepsia*, 1997, 38, 998-1007.

Baxendale, SA; Thompson, PJ; van Paesschen, W. A test of spatial memory and its clinical utility in the pre-surgical investigation of temporal lobe epilepspy patients. *Neuropsychologia*, 1998, 36, 591-602.

Beatty, WW. A strategy for studying memory disorders in multiple sclerosis. In: Squire RL, Butters N editors. *Neuropsychology of memory*. New York, NY: Guilford Press; 1992; 285-289.

Bechara, A; Tranel, D; Damasio, H; Adolphs, R; Rockland, C; Damasio, AR. Double dissociation of conditioning and declarative knowledge relative to the amygdala and hippocampus in humans. *Science*, 1995, 269, 1115-1118.

Beck, AT. *Beck Depression Inventory*. San Antonio, TX: The Psychological Corporation; 1987.

Benedict, RH; Munschauer, F; Linn, R; Miller, C; Murphy, E; Foley, F; Jacobs, L. Screening for multiple sclerosis cognitive impairment using a self-administered 15-item questionnaire. *Multiple Sclerosis*, 2003, 9, 95-101.

Benton, AL; Hamsher, KS; Varney, NR; Spreen, O. *Contributions to neuropsychological assessment*. New York, NY: Oxford University Press; 1983.

Bever, CT; Grattan, L; Panitch, HS; Johnson, KP. The brief repeatable battery of neuropsychological tests for multiple sclerosis: a preliminary serial study. *Multiple Sclerosis*, 1995, 1, 165-169.

Bohbot, VD; Kalina, M; Stepankova, K; Spackova, N; Petrides, M; Nadel, L. Spatial memory deficits in patients with lesions to the right hippocampus and to the right parahippocampal cortex. *Neuropsychologia*, 1998, 36, 1217-1238.

Boringa, JB; Lazeron, RH; Reuling, IE; Ader, HJ; Pfennings, L; Lindeboom, J; de Sonneville, LM; Kalkers, NF; Polman, CH. The brief repeatable battery of neuropsychological tests: normative values allow application in multiple sclerosis clinical practice. *Multiple Sclerosis*, 2001, 7, 263-267.

Caramazza, A. Is cognitive neuropsychology possible? *Journal of Cognitive Neuroscience*, 1992, 4, 80-95.

Cendes, F; Andermann, F; Dubeau, F; Gloor, P; Evans, A; Jones-Goatman, M; Olivier, A; Andermann, E; Robitaille, Y; Lopes-Cendes, I; Peters, T; Melanson, D. Early childhood prolonged febrile convulsions, atrophy and sclerosis of mesial structures, and temporal lobe epilepsy: an MRI volumetric study. *Neurology*, 1993a, 43, 1083-1087.

Cendes, F; Andermann, F; Gloor, P; Lopes-Cendes, I; Andermann, E; Melanson, D; Jones-Gotman, M; Robitaille, Y; Evans, A; Peters, T. Atrophy of mesial structures in patients with temporal lobe epilepsy: cause or consequence of repeated seizures? *Annals of Neurology*, 1993b, 34, 795-801.

Cendes, F; Kobayashi, E. Epilepsia de lobo temporal. In: Guerreiro CAM, Guerreiro MM, Cendes F, Lopes-Cendes I editors, *Epilepsia*. São Paulo: Lemos Editorial; 2000; 201-213.

Comi, G; Filippi, M; Barkhof, F; Durelli, L; Edan, G; Fernandez, O; Hartung, H; Seeldrayers, P; Sorensen, PS; Rovaris, M; Martinelli, V; Hommes, OR. Effect of early interferon treatment on conversion to definite multiple sclerosis: a randomized study. *Lancet*, 2001, 357, 1576-1582.

Crawford, JR; Garthwaite, PH. Investigation of the single case in neuropsychology: confidence limits on the abnormality of test scores and test score differences. *Neuropsychologia*, 2002, 40, 1196-1208.

Crawford, JR: Garthwaite, PH. Detecting dissociations in single-case studies: Type I errors, statistical power and the classical versus strong distinction. *Neuropspychologia*, 2006, 44, 2249-2258.

Crick, F. The recent excitement about neural networks. *Nature*, 1989, 337, 129-132.

Cutter, GC; Baier, ML; Rudick, RA; Cookfair, DL; Fischer, JS; Petkau, J; Syndulko, K; Weinshenker, BG; Antel, JP; Confavreux, C; Ellison, GW; Lublin, F; Miller, AE; Rao, SM; Reingold, S; Thompson, A; Willoughby, E. Development of a multiple sclerosis functional composite as a clinical trial outcome measure. *Brain*, 1999, 122, 871-882.

Damasceno, A; Delicio, AM; Mazo, DFC; Zullo, JFD; Scherer, P; Ng, RTY; Damasceno, BP. Validation of the Brazilian version of mini-test CASI-S. *Arq Neuropsiquiatr*, 2005, 63, 416-421.

Damasio, H; Damasio, AR. *Lesion analysis in neuropsychology*. New York, NY: Oxford University Press; 1989.

Damasio, H; Damasio, AR. The lesion method in behavioral neurology and neuropsychology. In: Feinberg TE, Farah MJ editors. *Behavioral neurology and neuropsychology*. New York, NY: McGraw-Hill Co.; 1997; 69-82.

Deloire, MS; Salort, E; Bonnet, M; Arimone, Y; Boudineau, M; Amieva, H; Barroso, B; Ouallet, JC; Pachai, C; Galliaud, E; Petry, KG; Dousset, V; Fabrigoule, C; Brochet, B. Cognitive impairment as marker of diffuse brain abnormalities in early relapsing remitting multiple sclerosis. *Journal of Neurology, Neurosurgery, and Psychiatry*, 2005, 76, 519-526.

Dennet, DC. *Consciousness explained*. Boston: Little, Brown and Co.; 1991.

De Renzi, E; Vignolo, LA. The Token test: a sensitive test to detect disturbances in aphasicis. *Brain*, 1962, 85, 665-678.

De Stefano, N; Narayanan, S; Francis, GS; Amaoutelis, R; Tartaglia, MC; Antel, JP; Matthews, PM; Arnold, DL. Evidence of axonal damage in the early stages of multiple sclerosis and its relevance to disability. *Archives of Neurology*, 2001, 58, 65-70.

Dronkers, NF. A new brain region for coordinating speech articulation. *Nature*, 1996, 384, 159-161.

Dronkers, NF; Redfern, BB; Knight, RT. The neural architecture of language disorders. In: Gazzaniga MS, editor. *The new cognitive neurosciences* (2nd edition). Cambridge, MA: The MIT Press; 2000; 949-958.

Engel, J; Willimson, PD; Wieser, HG. Mesial temporal lobe epilepsy. In: Engel J, Pendley TA editors. *Epilepsy: a comprehensive textbook*. Philadelphia: Lippincott-Raven Pyblishers; 1997; 2417-2426.

Folstein, MF; Folstein, SF; McHugh, PR. Mini-Mental State: a practical method for grading the cognitive state of patients for the clinician. *Journal of Psychiatric Research*, 1975, 12, 189-198.

Fuster, JM. *The prefrontal cortex: anatomy, physiology, and neuropsychology of the frontal lobe* (2nd edition). New York, NY: Raven Press; 1989.

Galperin, PY. *An introduction to psychology*. Moscow: Moscow University Press; 1976. (in Russian).

Gazzaniga, MS; Ivry, RB; Mangun, GR. *Cognitive neuroscience: the biology of the mind*. New York, NY: W.W. Norton and Co.; 1998.

Gazzaniga, MS; Ivry, RB; Mangun, GR. *Cognitive neuroscience: the biology of the mind* (2nd edition). New York, NY: W. W. Norton and Co.; 2002.

Gleissner, U; Helmstaedter, C; Schramm, J; Elger, CE. Memory outcome after selective amygdalo-hippocampectomy: a study in 140 patients with temporal lobe epilepsy. *Epilepsia*, 2002, 43, 87-95.

Golby, AJ; Poldrack, RA; Illes, J; Chen, D; Desmond, JE; Gabrieli, JDE. Memory lateralization in medial temporal lobe epilepsy assessed by functional MRI. *Epilepsia*, 2002, 43, 855-863.

Grant, CM; McDonald, WI; Trimble, MR; Smith, E; Reed, R. Deficient learning and memory in early and middle phases of multiple sclerosis. *Journal of Neurology, Neurosurgery, and Psychiatry*, 1984, 47, 250-255.

Hamann, S; Ely, T; Grafton, S; Kilts, C. Amygdala activity related to enhanced memory for pleasant and aversive stimuli. *Nature Neuroscience*, 1999, 2, 289-293.

Hart, J; Berndt, RS; Caramazza, A. Category-specific naming deficit following cerebral infarction. *Nature*, 1985, 316, 439-440.

Heaton, RK; Chelune, GJ; Talley, JL; Kay, GG; Curtiss, G. *Wisconsin Card Sorting test manual – revised and expanded*. USA: Psychological Assessment Resources; 1993.

Heinemann, U; Draguhn, A; Meierkord, H. The pathophysiology of seizure generation. In: Shorvon S, Dreifuss F, Fish D, Thomas D editors. *The treatment of epilepsy*. London: Blackwell Science; 1996.

Hermann, BP; Connell, B; Barr, WB; Wyler, AR. The utility of the Warrington Recognition Memory test for temporal lobe epilepsy: pre- and postoperative results. *Journal of Epilepsy*, 1995, 8, 139-145.

Hermann, BP; Seidenberg, M; Schoenfeld, J; Davies, K. Neuropsychological characteristics of the syndrome of mesial temporal lobe epilepsy. *Archives of Neurology*, 1997, 54, 369-376.

Hooper, HE. *Hooper visual organization test (VOT)*. Los Angeles: Western Psychological Services; 1983.

Huettel, SA; Song, AW; McCarthy, G. *Functional magnetic resonance imaging*. Sunderland, MA: Sinauer Associates, Inc.; 2004.

Jackson, JH. On the nature of the duality of the brain. In: *Selected writings of John Hughlings Jackson*. New York, NY: Basic Books; 1958.

Jacobs, LD; Beck, RW; Simon, JH; Kinkel, RP; Brownscheidle, CM; Murray, TJ; Simonian, NA; Slasor, PJ; Sandrock, AW. Intramuscular interferon beta-1a therapy initiated during a first demyelinating event in multiple sclerosis. CHAMPS Study Group. *New England Journal of Medicine*, 2000, 343, 898-904.

Jezzard, P; Matthews, PM; Smith, SM editors. *Functional MRI: an introduction to methods*.

Oxford: Oxford University Press; 2001.

Jones-Gotman, M. Psychological evaluation for epilepsy surgery. In: Shorvon S, Dreifuss F, Fish D, Thomas D editors. *The treatment of epilepsy*. Oxford: Blackwell Science; 1996; 621-630.

Jones-Gotman, M; Brulot, M; McMackin, D; Cendes, F; Andermann, F; Olivier, A; Evans, A; Peters, T. Word and design list learning deficits related to side of hippocampal atrophy as assessed by volumetric MRI measurements. *Epilepsia*, 1993, 34 (Suppl. 6), 71.

Jones-Gotman, M; Zatorre, RJ; Olivier, A; Andermann, F; Cendes, F; Staunton, H; McMackin, D; Siegel, AM; Wieser, H-G. Learning and retention of words and designs following excision from medial or lateral temporal lobe structures. *Neuropsychologia*, 1997, 35, 963-973.

Kaplan, EF; Goodglass, H; Weintraub, S. *Boston naming test* (2nd edition). Philadelphia: Lea and Febiger; 1983.

Kappos, L; Polman, CH; Freedman, MS; Edan, G; Hartung, HP; Miller, DH; Montalban, X; Barkhof, F; Bauer, L; Jacobs, P; Pohl, C; Sandbrink, R.Treatment with interferon beta-1b delays conversion to clinically definite and McDonald MS in patients with clinically isolated syndrome. *Neurology*, 2006, 67, 1242-1249.

Katzman, R; Brown, T; Fuld, P; Peck, A; Schechter, R; Schimmel, H. Validation of a short Orientation-memory-concentration test of cognitive impairment. *American Journal of Psychiatry*, 1983, 140, 734-739.

Kiehl, KA; Smith, AM; Mendrek, A; Forster, BB; Hare, RD; Liddle, PF. Activation of the amygdala during an affective memory task. *NeuroImage*, 1998, 7, S902.

Kinsbourne, M. Cognitive deficit: experimental analysis. In: McGaugh JL, editor. *Psychobiology*. New York, NY: Academic Press; 1971.

Kurtzke, JF. Rating neurologic impairment in multiple sclerosis: an expanded disability status scale (EDSS). *Neurology*, 1983, 33, 1444-1452.

Leischner, A. Über den Verlauf und die Einteilung der aphasischen Syndrome. *Archiv für Psychiatrie und Nervenkrankheiten*, 1972, 216, 219-231.

Leone, AAA; Damasceno, BP; Cendes, F; Guerreiro, CAM. Memory deficits in patients with temporal lobe epilepsy. *Journal of the International Neuropsychological Society*, 2001, 7, 429.

Leontiev, AN. *Problems of the development of the mind.* Moscow: Progress Publishers; 1981a.

Leontiev, AN. The problem of activity in psychology. In: Wertsch JV, editor. *The concept of activity in soviet psychology*. New York, NY: M. E. Sharpe; 1981b; 38-71.

Lezak, MD. *Neuropsychological assessment* (3rd edition). New York, NY: Oxford University Press; 1995.

Loring, DW; Meador, KJ. Neuropsychological assessment for epilepsy surgery. In: Feinberg TE, Farah MJ editors. *Behavioral neurology and neuropsychology*. New York, NY: McGraw-Hill; 1997; 657-666.

Luria, AR. *Higher cortical functions in man* (2nd edition). New York, NY: Basic Books; 1966/1980.

Luria, AR. *The working brain: an introduction to neuropsychology*. New York, NY: Basic Books; 1973.

Magaziner, J; Basset, SS; Hebel, JR. Predicting performance on the Mini-Mental State Examination. *Journal of the American Geriatrics Society*, 1987, 35, 996-1000.

McAlpine, D. The benign form of multiple sclerosis: results of a long-term study. *British Medical Journal*, 1964, 2, 1029-1032.

McDonald, WI; Compston, A; Edan, G; Goodkin, D; Hartung, HP; Lublin, FD; McFarland, HF; Patty, DW; Polman, CH; Reingold, SC; Sandberg-Wollheim, M; Sibley, W; Thompson, A; van den Noort,S; Weinshenker, BY; Wolinsky, JS. Recommended diagnostic criteria for multiple sclerosis: guidelines from the International Panel on the diagnosis of multiple sclerosis. *Annals of Neurology*, 2001, 50, 121-127).

Mesulam, M-M. Large-scale neurocognitive networks and distributed processing for attention, language, and memory. *Annals of Neurology*, 1990, 28, 597-613.

Milner, B. Psychological defects produced by temporal lobe excision. *Research Publications – Association for Research in Nervous and Mental Disease*,1958, 36, 244-257.

Milner, B. Interhemispheric differences in the localization of psychological processes in man. *British Medical Bulletin*, 1971, 27, 272-277.

Novelly, RA; Williamson, PD. Incidence of false-positive memory impairment in the intracarotid amytal procedure. *Epilepsia*, 1989, 30, 711.

O'Keefe, J; Nadel, L. *The hippocampus as a cognitive map*. Oxford: Clarendon Press; 1978.

Okuda, B; Tanaka, H; Tachibana, H; Iwamoto, Y; Takeda, M; Kawabata, K; Sugita, M. Visual form agnosia in multiple sclerosis. *Acta Neurologica Scandinavica*, 1996, 94, 38-44.

Osterrieth, PA. Le test de copie d´une figure complexe. *Archives de Psychologie*, 1944, 30, 206-356.

Pelosi, L; Geesken, JM; Holly, M; Hayward, M; Blumhardt, LD. Working memory impairment in early multiple sclerosis: evidence from an event-related potential study of patients with clinically isolated myelopathy. *Brain*, 1997, 120, 2039-2058.

Peyser, JM; Rao, SM; LaRocca, NG; Kaplan, E. Guidelines for neuropsychological research in multiple sclerosis. *Archives of Neurology*, 1990, 47, 94-97.

Phillips, ML; Young, AW; Scott, SK; Calder, AJ; Andrew, C; Giampietro, V; Williams, SC; Bullmore, ET; Brammer, M; Gray, JA. Neural responses to facial and vocal expressions of fear and disgust. *Proceedings of the Royal Society of London. B: Biological Sciences*, 1998, 265, 1809-1817.

Rao, SM. Neuropsychological aspects of multiple sclerosis. In: Raine CS, McFarland HF, Tourtellotte WW editors. *Multiple sclerosis: clinical and pathogenetic basis*. London, England: Chapman and Hall; 1997; 357-362.

Rao, SM; Leo, GJ; Bernardin, L; Unverzagt, F. Cognitive dysfunction in multiple sclerosis: I. Frequency, patterns, and prediction. *Neurology*, 1991, 41, 685-691.

Rey, A. *L´examen clinique en psychologie*. Paris: Presses Universitaires de France; 1964.

Rovaris, M; Filippi, M; Falautano, M; Minicucci, L; Rocca, MA; Martinelli, V; Comi, G. Relation between MR abnormalities and patterns of cognitive impairment in multiple sclerosis. *Neurology*, 1998, 50, 1601-1608.

Rovaris, M; Comi, G; Filippi, M. MRI markers of destructive pathology in multiple sclerosis-related cognitive dysfuction. *Journal of Neurological Sciences*; 2006, 245, 111-116.

Rummelhart, DE; McClelland JL. *Parallel distributed processing: explorations in the microstructure of cognition*. Cambridge, MA: MIT Press; 1986.

Sass, KJ; Lencz, T; Westerveld, M; Novelly, RA; Spencer, DD; Kim, JH. The neural substrate of memory impairment demonstrated by the intracarotid amobarbital procedure. *Archives of Neurology*, 1991, 48, 48-52.

Sbordone, RJ; Long, CJ. *Ecological validity of neuropsychological testing.* Delray Beach, FL: GR Press / St. Lucie Press; 1996.

Shallice, T. *From neuropsychology to mental structure*. Cambridge: Cambridge University Press; 1988.

Smith, ML; Milner, B. The role of the right hippocampus in the recall of spatial location. *Neuropsychologia*, 1981, 19, 781-793.

Stroop, JR. Studies of interference in serial verbal reactions. *Journal of Experimental Psychology*, 1935, 18, 643-662.

Suzuki, WA; Zola-Morgan, S; Squire, LR; Amaral, DG. Lesions of the perirhinal and parahippocampal cortices in the monkey produce long-lasting memory impairment in the visual and tactual modalities. *Journal of Neuroscience*, 1993, 13, 2430-2451.

Swirsky-Sacchetti, T; Field, HL; Mitchell, DR; Seward, J; Lublin, FD; Knobler, RL; Gonzalez, CF. The sensitivity of the Mini-Mental State Exam in the white matter dementia of multiple sclerosis. *Journal of Clinical Psychology*, 1992, 48, 779-786.

Tabert, MH; Borod, JC; Tang, CY; Lange, G; Wei, TC; Johnson, R; Nusbaum, AO; Buchsbaum, MS. Differential amygdala activation during emotional decision and recognition memory tasks using unpleasant words: an fMRI study. *Neuropsychologia*, 2001, 39, 556-573.

Tellez-Zenteno, JF; Dhar, R; Hernandez-Ronquillo, L; Wiebe, S. Long-term outcomes in epilepsy surgery: antiepileptic drugs, mortality, cognitive and psychosocial aspects. *Brain* (in press).

Teng, EL; Larson, EB; Lin, KN; Graves, AB; Liu, HC. Screening for dementia: the Cognitive Abilities Screening Instrument - Short Version (CASI-Short). Paper presented at the Annual Convention of the American Psychological Association, San Francisco, 1998.

Teuber, HL. Physiological psychology. *Annual Review of Psychology*, 1955, 9, 267-296.

Tomasello, M; Kruger, AC; Ratner, HH. Cultural learning. *Behavioral and Brain Sciences*, 1993, 16, 495-552.

Trenerry, MR; Jack, CR; Ivnik, RJ; Sharbrough, FW; Cascino, GD; Hirschorn, KA; Marsh, WR; Kelly, PJ; Meyer, FB. MRI hippocampal volumes and memory function before and after temporal lobectomy. *Neurology*, 1993, 43, 1800-1805.

Von Monakow, C. *Über Lokalisation der Hirnfunktionen*. Wiesbaden: Von Bergmann; 1910.

Vygotsky, LS. *Mind in society: the development of higher psychological processes*. Cambridge, MA: Harvard University Press; 1978.

Vygotsky, LS. Psychology and the theory of localization of psychic functions. In: Vygotsky LS, editor. *Sobranie sochinenij. Tom 1. Voprosy teorii i istorii psikhologii*. Moscow: Pedagogika; 1934/1982; 168-174. (in Russian)

Webster's Comprehensive Dictionary of the English Language. Naples, FL: Trident Press International; 1996.

Wechsler, D. *Wechsler Adult Intelligence Scale – Revised*. New York, NY: The Psychological Corporation; 1981.

Wechsler, D. *Wechsler Memory Scale – Revised: manual*. San Diego: Psychological Corporation / Harcourt Brace Jovanovich; 1987.

Weiskrantz, L. Some traps and pontifications. In: Weiskrantz L, editor. *Analysis of behavioral change*. New York, NY: Harper and Row; 1968.

Wertsch, JV. *Mind as action*. New York, NY: Oxford University Press; 1998.

Wiebe, S; Blume, WT; Girvin, JP; Eliasziw, M. A randomized, controlled trial of surgery for temporal-lobe epilepsy. *New England Journal of Medicine*, 2001, 345, 311-318.

Wilde, N; Strauss, E; Chelune, GJ; Loring, DW; Martin, RC; Hermann, BP; Sherman, E; Hunter, M. WMS-III performance in patients with temporal lobe epilepsy: group differences and individual classification. *Journal of the International Neuropsychological Society*, 2001, 7, 881-891.

In: Leading-Edge Cognitive Disorders Research
Editor: James P. Tsai, pp. 155-167
ISBN: 978-1-60021-843-9

Chapter 6

CHILD MOLESTERS' COGNITIVE DISTORTIONS: A BRIEF RESEARCH REVIEW

Siân E. Williams[a], Theresa A. Gannon[b1], Tony Ward[c], and Rachael M. Collie[c]
[a]Canterbury Christchurch University, UK
[b]University of Kent, UK
[c]Victoria University of Wellington, New Zealand

ABSTRACT

There are few criminal offences capable of stirring up as much public anger and disgust as child molestation. Despite the media fuelled public perception that child molesters (CMs) cannot be treated, research into the cognition of CMs is suggesting that we may be able to challenge some of the belief structures of these individuals and thus change their behavior patterns. Attempts to discover why some people molest children are paramount to delivering effective treatment programs. In this chapter, we will provide an overview of the main research methodologies and theories that have been developed over the past two decades to investigate the cognitive distortions of CMs and consider how empirical research may inform treatment programs.

It is perhaps not surprising that the cognition of CMs (i.e., what they think and believe), has become central to both research and treatment programs over the last two decades since virtually all contemporary theories of child molestation highlight the importance of cognition (e.g., Finkelhor, 1984; Hall and Hirschman, 1992; Ward and Siegert, 2002). The role of cognitive distortions in particular has been suggested as fundamental to the etiology and treatment of child sexual abuse. The underlying assumption is that CMs' thinking is distorted or different from non-molesters in distinct and important ways. It is these distortions in thinking that we intend to focus upon in this chapter.

[1] Address for chapter correspondence: Dr. Theresa Gannon, Keynes College University of Kent, Canterbury CT1 7NP. E-Mail: *T.A.Gannon@Kent.ac.uk*, Phone: +44 (0)1227 824 827, Fax: +44 (0) 1227 827 030.

WHAT ARE COGNITIVE DISTORTIONS?

Broadly speaking, the term *cognitive distortion* (CD) is often used to refer to a systematic thinking pattern that is in some way biased or untrue (e.g., Beck, 1963, 1967, 1976, 1987; Rachman and Shafran, 1999). We are complex beings: we do not simply react to our social worlds, we selectively attend to some events and ignore others; we place our own interpretation on others' behaviors and situations; and we respond accordingly to that *interpretation* rather than the actual event. People with CDs are, therefore, often responding to misinterpretations of an event. CDs have been associated with many mental disorders such as depression (e.g. Beck, Rush and Shaw, 1979), obsessive-compulsive disorder (e.g. Salkovskis, 1985), anorexia and bulimia (e.g. Garner and Bemis, 1982; Thompson, Berg and Shatford, 1987), and underpin many successful treatment programs in the shape of Cognitive-Behavioral Therapy.

The term *cognitive distortion* was first used in the sexual offending literature when Gene Abel and his colleagues applied the concept to CMs (see Abel, Becker, and Cunningham-Rathner, 1984). Despite many vagaries in definitions over the past two decades (see Gannon, Ward and Collie, 2006 or Maruna and Mann, in press), some researchers define the term CDs (Gannon and Polaschek, in press) using the *cognitive distortion hypothesis*. This hypothesis states that convicted CMs hold relatively well-established and generalized offense-related beliefs that facilitate sexually abusive behavior (see Abel, Gore, Holland, Camp, Becker and Rathner, 1989; Beech and Mann, 2002; Bumby, 1996; Mann and Beech, 2003; Saradjian and Nobus, 2003; Ward, 2000; Ward and Keenan, 1999). It is this deliberately focused definition that we intend to use throughout this chapter, since to talk of all the possible mechanisms driving CMs' cognition would be prohibitive within our space constraints.

The exact development and nature of CMs' distorted beliefs is a matter of some debate but it is generally hypothesized that some CMs misinterpret the innocent behavior of children as being somehow sexual and they react to that misinterpretation rather than a rational or true appraisal of the situation (Mann and Shingler, 2006; Ward, 2000).

The idea that CMs may have a belief-system that differs from non-CMs is embedded in a social-cognitive framework (Ward, Hudson, Johnston, and Marshall, 1997). Social cognition is concerned with how each of us uniquely experiences and makes sense of our social world (Fiske and Taylor, 1991). It is argued that to understand any given behavior we must consider the *content* and *structure* of knowledge stored in memory, how this effects the *processing* of social information, and how these existing structures may be modified (Sherman, Judd, and Park, 1989). So in relation to child molestation the aim is to investigate the content of offense-supportive knowledge and how this is structured in memory, how this information effects the interpretation of information such as children's actions and behaviors, and how treatment may address changing these belief structures.

INVESTIGATING CHILD MOLESTERS' COGNITIVE DISTORTIONS

Elucidating the existence and then the nature of CMs' CDs poses a real challenge for researchers in the field. It is not possible to 'look inside someone's head' to see what they are thinking. Instead methodologies have to be developed to gain access to the thought processes of the CM. In this section we will present a brief overview of the main methodologies employed in this area over the past twenty years (for a more extensive review see Gannon and Polaschek, in press). The first two we shall look at are very direct methods which require the CM to reflect on their thinking patterns. The third uses more indirect methods designed to avoid self-presentation biases and the problems associated with self-reflection.

TAPPING COGNITIVE PRODUCTS

Analysis of Post Offence Statements

If we want to understand the thought processes that lead a CM to commit their crime perhaps a good place to start is to ask the individual why they did it. Hollon and Kriss (1984) suggested that asking individuals about their behaviors may reveal glimpses into their entire cognitive system (i.e., their cognitive content, structures, and processes). They use the term *cognitive products* to describe the outcome of interactions between cognitive content, structures, and processing.

Cognitive Products were first formally investigated by Abel et al. (1984) who analyzed CMs' post-offense statements. Although their exact method is unclear they appear to have drawn on their clinical experience with CMs in order to categorize and describe some typical CM beliefs. Abel et al. extracted seven categories of beliefs: a) a lack of physical resistance from a child means they are a willing sexual partner, (b) being sexual with children educates them about sex, (c) children don't tell others about sexual abuse because they like it, (d) mere fondling of children won't really harm them, (e) children ask about sex because they want to be shown it, (f) having sex with children brings the adult and child closer together, and (g) society will learn to accept child-adult sexual relationships in the future.

This work was an interesting starting point. However it appeared that there was much more room for categorization. Over the next few years, some researchers compiled additional lists of offence-supportive cognition (e.g., Neidigh and Krop, 1992; Pollock and Hashmall, 1991). Neidigh and Krop (1992), for instance, document an extensive database of CMs post-offense statements from a questionnaire that they distributed to 101 CMs designed to identify the "thoughts, ideas or beliefs" (p. 210) that CMs believed contributed to their offense. From this database Neidigh and Krop identified 38 categories of beliefs. While some of these categories were consistent with the findings of Abel et al. (1984) some additional categories were suggested (e.g. "I was high on drugs and alcohol at the time", "I wasn't thinking at all or I wouldn't have done it").

While studies of this type can be in useful in providing some insight into the offense-supportive beliefs of CMs and have been used to develop more standardized measures (discussed in more detail below) the value of these descriptive lists should perhaps be questioned. One important consideration is whether the statements CMs produce regarding their offences are reflective of an underlying belief system or whether they are simply post-hoc justifications. Using this type of methodology there really is no way of knowing what is motivating CMs' post-offence justificatory statements. This is an important consideration with real theoretical and practical implications: lists of distorted statements do little to advance our conceptual understanding of CMs' cognition and thus offer limited guidance for theory or treatment.

Despite these limitations early methodology really did open up the field for researchers interested in CMs' cognition. Abel's work kick-started inquiry into previously untouched areas and the results of such studies provided a starting point from which to focus more standardized methodologies such as psychometric methods.

Psychometric Analysis of Cognitive Distortions

A second popular method for studying the cognition of CMs has been to use questionnaires. These CD scales are usually developed from CMs' statements (cognitive products) about their own offences and often contain individualized offense supportive statements (e.g. "I show my love and affection to a child by having sex with her [him]") and general offense supportive statements (e.g. "when a young child has sex with an adult, it helps the child learn how to relate to adults in the future"; Abel et al., 1989). Typically respondents are asked to read a list of statements and then indicate on a Likert scale the extent to which they agree with each of them. These are administered to CMs and their responses are compared with various non-CM comparison groups. If CMs really do hold distorted beliefs then we should be able to distinguish them from men who do not molest children based on their responses to these questionnaires (Ward et al., 1997).

A number of these cognitive distortion scales exist in the literature (for a review see Vanhouche and Vertommen, 1999). They differ in the exact number and nature of the CDs on the questionnaire and in the response scale used (i.e., some use Likert scales strongly disagree–strongly agree while others use a true-false format). Two widely used scales are the Abel and Becker Cognitions Scale (ABCS; Abel et al., 1989) and the MOLEST scale (Bumby, 1996). Let us examine these two scales and some research using them.

The ABCS contains 29 statements such as "When a young child has sex with an adult, it helps the child learn how to relate to adults in the future". Respondents are asked to read each statement and indicate the extent to which they agree with each on a five-point Likert scale. Scores for each statement are summed across the full questionnaire and then CMs' total scores are compared with the comparison group(s). Work with the ABCS has found that it can successfully discriminate CMs from community controls (Abel et al., 1989; Stermac and Segal, 1989; Tierney and McCabe, 2001), rapists (Stermac and Segal, 1989), and non-CM offenders[2] (Hayashino, Wurtle, and Klebe, 1995), however some studies have not reported successful discriminations between CMs and non-CM offenders (e.g. Abel et al., 1989; Tierney and McCabe, 2001). Where discrimination is found it indicates that CMs have scores higher on the scale overall suggesting more CD endorsement (a point we will return to shortly).

Another popularly used scale is Bumby's (1996) MOLEST scale. The MOLEST scale contains 38 items rated using a 4-point scale. Studies using this scale have found it can significantly discriminate CMs from rapists (Arkowitz and Vess, 2003; Bumby, 1996), non-CM offenders (Bumby, 1996; Marshall, Marshall, Sachdev, and Kruger, 2003); and

[2] The statistical discrimination held for extra-familial CMs but not for intra-familial CMs.

community comparisons (Marshall et al., 2003). In addition the scores on the MOLEST have been found to correlate with the number of victims in CMs' offense histories (Bumby, 1996).

The results from studies using such cognitive distortion scales are fairly mixed and even when a scale does discriminate CMs from the non-CMs we have to consider the clinical, as well as the statistical, significance of the result. A closer examination of the results of such studies often shows that CMs do not agree with the statements. To explain, they tend to disagree with the statements but tend to do so less vehemently than the non-CM controls allowing for statistically significant differences to be found. So while in interviews CMs seem to be producing many distorted cognitive products, in questionnaire studies similar statements do not appear to be endorsed.

There is some concern over the extent to which CMs are responding truthfully to scales such as the ABCS and the MOLEST. For instance it has been suggested that the statements forming the scale are likely to elicit socially desirable responding (Langevin, 1991; McGrath, Cann, and Konopasky, 1998; Murphy, 1990; Vanhouche and Vertommen, 1999). The worry is that CMs know how they should respond to the statements (especially if they have gone through or are going through some program of treatment) and respond in a socially desirable way rather than revealing their true thoughts. This could explain why CD endorsements are so low; CMs are simply hiding their unsavory beliefs from professionals.

In a recent effort to test this hypothesis, Gannon (2002, 2006) experimentally manipulated propensity to respond honestly by hooking CMs up to a 'lie-detector'. The results from this study showed that, despite a reasonably high belief that the lie-detector could detect lies CMs (both treated and untreated) were no more likely to endorse the cognitive products when attached to the detector than when they were not. In a similar study conducted with untreated CMs (Gannon, Keown, and Polaschek, 2006), despite a significant increase in item endorsement scores, CMs were no more likely to agree with the statements under the lie-detector condition than they were under the standard pen and paper condition.

In summary, psychometric methods offer a practical way of assessing CDs in treatment and research. However they should be used with an appreciation of the issues and limitations associated with them. Namely that they rely on self-report honesty and that they assume that CM respondents can accurately access and retrieve their belief structures (which Gannon's studies suggest may not be the case).

Tapping Cognitive Processing

More recently, researchers have begun looking to mainstream cognitive psychology to provide more sophisticated methods for assessing what goes on in the CM's mind. The methods are based on the assumption that information and knowledge is represented in the mind in structured ways. Concepts and knowledge are connected in our long-term memories based on our experiences in the world. These 'knowledge structures' influence our perception of events as well our reaction to them and our memory of them.

By looking at how CMs process the information they encounter, for example how they perceive it, how they interpret it, and how they remember it, we may begin to understand how they structure it and see if these knowledge structures are any different to comparison groups. These methodologies avoid the problem of participant introspection and social desirability associated with questionnaires and interviews as they do not explicitly require CMs to make introspective judgments.

Research in this area is relatively new but promising. A few studies have sought to investigate the specific concepts that CMs associate with children using what is known as the Implicit Association Task (IAT; Greenwald, McGee, and Schwartz, 1998; see also Mihailides, Devilly and Ward, 2004; Gray, Brown, MacCulloch, Smith and Snowdon, 2005). The IAT is designed to tap unconscious associations that an individual may hold between concepts by recording response times to paired words. Faster response times are believed to reflect stronger mental associations for the individual. CMs taking part in these types of studies are typically presented with cognitive distortion congruent pairings such as children and sex words as well cognitive distortion incongruent pairings such as children and non-sex words. Results from such studies have suggested that CMs do indeed associate children with sexual concepts (Milhailides el al., 2004; Gray et al., 2005). It could be argued however that these studies merely illustrate that CMs are more familiar with such concepts because they are required to talk about them more (e.g., during forensic assessments, or as part of sexual offender treatment programs).

Traditional cognitive techniques have also been employed recently to test the assertion that CMs intentionally respond in socially desirable ways or 'fake good' on psychometric measures of CDs. Based on the finding that faking good is associated with faster response times in comparison to honest responses (e.g., Hsu, Santelli and Hsu, 1989) Gannon and Polaschek (2005) recorded CMs' response times to CDs and to statements that should not tempt dishonest responding (i.e., control beliefs such as "The date we were born on is usually called a birthday"). In comparing CMs' responses with offender and non-offender comparisons they found that that treated CMs did endorse less CDs than non-treated CMs (consistent with the hypothesis that treatment modifies CMs' cognition) but also that they responded faster than the untreated CMs and the comparison groups. The authors suggest that this reaction time difference may indicate that CMs are faking good post-treatment: a finding that would otherwise be inaccessible through traditional interview and questionnaire methodologies.

Other researchers have provided CMs with rather transparent 'vignettes' of child-adult sexual interaction of varying degrees of severity followed up with questions designed to investigate how the story has been perceived and interpreted. These studies have found that unless the behavior of the child is unambiguously negative (i.e. crying) CMs (in comparison to comparison groups) report the child to enjoy the experience more, and to hold more responsibility for the abuse (Stermac and Segal, 1989). These findings appear to suggest that CMs may make self-serving perceptions of children's behavior.

Other work with vignettes has looked at the automatic interpretations of CMs by examining their memory for an ambiguous story that ends in sexual abuse (Gannon, Wright, Beech, and Williams, 2006). While CM and the non-CM offender comparison group tended to recall the vignette incorrectly, and introduced a number of errors into their recall, neither group were particularly likely to reinterpret the stories using offense-related beliefs. In other words, it did not look at though these CMs used offense-related beliefs to interpret the vignette that they had read.

Research Methods: Conclusion

The main methodologies employed to investigate the cognition of CMs over the past two decades have employed interviews and questionnaire methods. Results from such studies have been fairly mixed with the interview data strongly suggesting that CMs hold a range of CDs but the questionnaire data suggesting that CMs rarely openly agree with such distorted thinking. More recently we have seen a surge of innovative techniques designed to tap the underlying cognitive processes of CMs. The results from these studies provide only partial support for the idea that CMs have distorted offense-supportive belief-structures. It may be that our current methods are simply not sophisticated enough to detect offence-supportive beliefs, or that offence-supportive beliefs do not exist as widely in CMs as the literature would suggest. Since newer research methodologies remain in their infancy, it may be some time before the full picture becomes clear.

From Data to Theoretical Explanations

The data shows that CMs talk about their own offences in ways that appear to support the cognitive distortion hypothesis. They sound as though they hold a range of offense-supportive beliefs. Let us now turn to looking at explanations for where these beliefs may come from and how they may be structured within the minds of CMs.

There are two prominent theories specific to CMs' CDs in the literature: Abel's *early theory* (e.g., 1984, 1989), and Ward's *implicit theories* (ITs; Ward, 2000; Ward and Keenan, 1999). They both focus on the idea that CMs hold distorted belief structures. However, they differ in the level of detail that they go into and in the explanation they offer for how CDs develop.

Abel and his colleagues provided the first theoretical account of CDs describing them within a Social Learning Theory framework. They suggested that in normal development boys learn to inhibit inappropriate sexual urges as they learn that society does not tolerate such behavior. These societal values and beliefs become integrated into the boy's own belief system. A small number of boys, for reasons not explicated by the theory, fail to learn to inhibit these urges and instead face a discord between the values of society and their own urges. To reduce this discord it is suggested that they reinterpret situations and the behaviors of others so that their own thoughts and actions begin to seem more appropriate or acceptable. This, according to Abel et al. (1989), is how CDs develop. Although not explicitly discussed in the original work this idea of reducing discord has been linked to 'cognitive dissonance' (Festinger, 1957) by Gannon and Polaschek (in press).

Abel's theory opened up new avenues of research into why some individuals molest children. For the first time researchers were looking at the cognition of CMs and coming up with viable suggestions as to why it differed from the cognition of non-CMs. It also had a huge impact on treatment where attention turned to the modification of CDs held by CMs.

This early theory focuses on a 'maintenance' role for offense-related beliefs in CMs: that CMs create CDs in order to reduce the conflict between their sexual urges and a societal belief system. However, the story does not end here. Abel's work was influential but leaves many unanswered questions. For example, why do some boys not learn to inhibit inappropriate sexual urges? Are the beliefs that CMs have specific to a certain situation/victim or are they more general beliefs as Abel's later use of the generalized questionnaire method implies (Gannon and Polaschek, in press)?

It was not until some 15 years later that Abel's theory was challenged by another significant theory. Ward (2000; Ward and Keenan, 1999) offered a theory of CDs that specifically outlines the types of beliefs that CMs may hold allowing researchers to specifically test the cognitive distortion hypothesis more directly. In short, Ward hypothesizes that CMs develop theories of their social world, based on their own experiences, which are offense-supportive. In childhood, before any offending has begun, Ward argues that these theories may be adaptive for the child. For example, a child who is physically beaten by his parents may learn to avoid adults believing them to be dangerous. However this theory if carried through to adulthood becomes maladaptive when the individual avoids adult contact preferring instead the company of children.

From the results of questionnaire and interview studies such as those outlined previously, Ward hypothesized that CMs may have one or more of five *implicit theories* (ITs). These are: children as sexual beings, nature of harm, dangerous world, entitlement, and uncontrollability.

Children as sexual beings. This IT holds that children enjoy sexual contact even with adults. It is hypothesized that CMs holding this IT interpret a child's innocent behavior in a sexually biased way. For example, a child showing affection such as wanting to hold hands may be interpreted by the CM as displaying sexually inviting behavior.

Nature of harm. This IT has two variants: one which holds that sexual acts are not harmful and the other that holds that only physically aggressive acts are harmful. A CM holding the first variant of the IT is likely to downplay society's concerns over sexual relations with children believing it to be harmless. A CM holding the second variant of the IT may believe that sexual relations with children are only harmful if it involves some physically aggressive act such as tying the child up. Both trivialize the harm involved in molestation.

Dangerous world. There are two variants of this IT based on the degree of danger the CM sees in his social world. CMs holding this IT are likely to see the world as excessively hostile and full of individuals who are out to exploit or reject them. CMs holding the less extreme version of this IT are likely to see children as the only safe haven in a dangerous world and so seek contact with them. CMs holding the more extreme version of this IT believe that children are also hostile and rejecting and may try to deal with them through sexual abuse and control.

Entitlement. This IT allows the CM to believe that his needs are more important than the needs of 'less worthy' individuals. Thus the CM holding this IT will feel entitled to fulfill his sexual needs with children whenever the urge takes him.

Uncontrollability. This IT exerts the belief that humans are out of control and one cannot control ones urges when more powerful forces are at play. Examples of these other forces are sexual urges, alcohol and drugs. A CM holding this IT will believe that his behavior was not in his control.

Ward (2000) theorized that a CM may hold one or many of these five ITs. Whereas Abel focused on the maintenance role of offense-supportive beliefs Ward et al. focus on their etiological role. The main assumption here is that the ITs exist before the offending begins and are fundamental to the offending starting.

A recent extension of Ward's original IT theory—the *Judgment Model of Cognitive Distortions*— has been offered by Ward, Gannon and Keown (2006). In brief, the model posits that CMs are likely to hold maladaptive values that accompany their ITs and that these ultimately provide the *driving force* for actions. In other words, maladaptive values may help to explain how ITs get translated into sexual offending behavior. The JMCD is a very recent theory and so there is no data specifically testing it to draw on at present.

The two prominent theories described all hold that distorted belief structures sit at the core of offending. While Abel opened up research and thinking on CMs' CDs, he did not adequately define what they were thus rendering research into them difficult and inconsistent. Ward's IT theory provided a much more concrete (although perhaps narrow) conception of CDs allowing researchers to test them more directly. It should be noted, however, that although interview data and IAT tasks appear to support the IT theory (e.g., Gray et al., 2005; Marziano, Ward, Beech, and Pattison, 2005; Mihailides et al., 2004), other experimental tasks have been unable to provide support for this theory (e.g., Gannon et al., 2006).

Applying Current Knowledge to Treatment

So how does all of the previously discussed information feed back into practice? One would certainly hope that there are some strong links with practice since the overarching aim of treatment should be to provide practice based on empirical evidence (McGuire, 2001). This section will provide a brief overview of how the theory and research covered in this section fits in with current treatment programs.

The early work of Abel and colleagues identified the distorted nature of CMs' belief systems. The lists of offence-supportive beliefs resulting from such work along with the discriminative ability of CD questionnaires were enough to convince treatment providers that a central part of any treatment package for CMs should be addressing CDs.

Abel's theory, however, left much open to interpretation. His conceptualization of what CDs were and their role in maintaining offending could be understood differently by different treatment providers. Furthermore, treatment efforts informed by Abel's theory centered on the victim-specific beliefs held by offenders since Abel's theory made no reference to the possible structure of offence-supportive beliefs in long-term memory. The specificity of Wards IT theory allowed for treatment to become more standardized and it encouraged a focus on challenging CMs' core schemas rather than victim-specific beliefs. In fact, many researchers are now taking a schema-based stance to understand CDs and how they should be treated, although not all programs specifically use Ward's (2000) particular schemas (see Beech and Mann, 2002; Drake, Ward, Nathan and Lee, 2001; Mann and Beech, 2003; Mann and Shingler, 2006). The use of schema-focused treatment programs is currently being adopted for offenders who appear to hold high levels of offense-supportive attitudes and does appear to add some value over and above the standard treatment package (Thornton and Shingler, 2001). However, research into the efficacy of such treatment programs is still relatively rare and is in need of further investigation.

Clearly then, treatment efforts do appear to have been informed by CD theory; but this does not necessarily mean that treatment is adequately informed by empirical research. Recall, that neither Abel nor Ward's theory is fully empirically supported at this time, since the development of quality research to test each theory's propositions has been rather slow. Given this fact, we believe that treatment providers should be aware that not all CMs may hold offence-supportive beliefs, as current manual based treatment programs would suggest

(Gannon, Polaschek, and Ward, 2005). Treating all CMs as though they hold offence-supportive schemas could be a dangerous assumption to make given the current lack of empirical evidence in this arena. Until we know more about this, therapists should try to keep mindful of the range of mechanisms that may produce offence-supportive statements since not all will be belief-based (see Maruna and Mann, in press, for an excellent discussion of such issues). For example, teaching CMs about their "thinking errors" or "distortions" if they are actually uttering post-hoc justifications may compromise both the therapist's credibility as well as the CM's motivation.

Future Directions and Conclusions

In this chapter we have seen some of the methodological and theoretical developments that have taken place over the past 20 years and we have considered how these have shaped treatment programs. So where do we go from here? What developments do we imagine we will see in this field over the next twenty years?

Firstly, let's consider the methodology used to elicit the CDs of CMs. In this chapter we have seen how interview and questionnaire designs allowed us to gain some grasp on how CMs explained their offenses but told us little about the mechanisms generating these explanations. It is suggested that future research may look to use interview methods alongside some more sophisticated methods designed to tap unconscious cognition (for example IAT studies). This may provide professionals with some more information around the mechanisms driving offence-supportive statements. For example, if CMs utter many explanatory statements during interview but then do not display offence-supportive associations on the IAT this may suggest that a good proportion of their 'distortions' are post-offence justifications. There is also more room to further explore questionnaire studies. In short, questionnaire studies rarely look at response patterns as a function of offender characteristics (e.g. treated versus untreated) or context (truly anonymous versus parole assessment). Examining these factors would perhaps provide a wider database of norms for researchers to work with and would also suggest the optimum conditions needed for best practice questionnaire assessment of CDs.

On the theoretical front we have seen some differences between, and sometimes within, the theories concerning the nature of offense-related beliefs. Research rarely explicates the theory it is designed to test. As such it is impossible to compare the relative value of the theories. Future research should be designed to explicitly test the propositions made by each of the proposed theories. It is anticipated that as more work with the theories is carried out there will be more opportunity to build an integrated and comprehensive theory of CMs' distorted cognition.

Treatment programs have progressed despite the lack of conceptual clarity and theoretical cohesion surrounding CMs belief structures. However it is important that future developments in treatment programs be informed by empirical work and not by intuition. After twenty years of research into the cognitive distortion hypothesis it is time for research to explicitly test the available theories so that we can begin to see *true* empirically driven practice in the cognitive arena.

REFERENCES

Abel, G. G., Becker, J. V., and Cunningham-Rathner, J. (1984). Complications, consent and cognitions in sex between children and adults. *International Journal of Law and Psychiatry, 7*,189-103.

Abel, G. G., Gore, D. K., Holland, C. L., Camp, N., Becker, J. V., and Rathner, J. (1989). The measurement of the cognitive distortions of child molesters. *Annals of Sex Research, 2*, 135-153.

Arkowitz, S., and Vess, J. (2003). An evaluation of the Bumby RAPE and MOLEST scales as measures of cognitive distortions with civilly committed sexual offenders. *Sexual Abuse: A Journal of Research and Treatment, 15*, 237-249.

Beck, A. T. (1963). Thinking and depression: 1. Idiosyncratic content and cognitive distortions. *Archives of General Psychiatry, 9,* 324-333.

Beck, A. T. (1967). *Depression: Clinical, experimental and theoretical aspects*. NY: Hoeber.

Beck, A. T. (1976). *Cognitive therapy and the emotional disorders*. NY: International Universities Press.

Beck, A. T. (1987). Cognitive models of depression. *Journal of Cognitive Psychotherapy, An International Quarterly, 1*, 5-37.

Beck, A. T., Rush, A. J., Shaw, B., *et al* (1979) *Cognitive Therapy of Depression.* NY: Wiley.

Beech, A. R., and Mann, R. (2002). Recent developments in the assessment and treatment of sexual offenders. In J. McGuire (Ed.), *Offender rehabilitation and treatment: Effective programmes and policies to reduce re-offending* (pp. 259-288). Chichester, UK: Wiley.

Bumby, K. M. (1996). Assessing the cognitive distortions of child molesters and rapists: Developments and validation of the MOLEST and RAPE scales. *Sexual Abuse: A Journal of Research and Treatment, 8*, 37-54.

Drake, C., Ward, T., Nathan, P, and Lee, J. (2001). Challenging the cognitive distortions of child molesters: An implicit theory approach. *Journal of Sexual Aggression, 7*, 25-40.

Festinger, L. (1957). *A Theory of Cognitive Dissonance*. Stanford, CA: Stanford University Press.

Finkelhor, D. (1984). *Child sexual abuse: New theory and research.* NY: Free Press.

Fiske, S. T., and Taylor, S. E. (1991). *Social cognition* (2nd ed.). NY: McGraw-Hill.

Gannon, T. A. (2002). *Cognitive distortions in child sexual offenders: Fact or fiction?* Unpublished doctoral dissertation, University of Sussex, Brighton, UK.

Gannon, T. A. (2006). Increasing honest responding on cognitive distortions in child molesters: The bogus pipeline procedure. *Journal of Interpersonal Violence, 21,* 1-18.

Gannon, T. A., Keown, K., and Polaschek (2006). The bogus pipeline with child molesters revisited. *Manuscript submitted for publication.*

Gannon, T. A., and Polaschek, D. L. L. (in press). Cognitive distortions in child molesters: A re-examination of key theories and research. *Clinical Psychology Review.*

Gannon, T. A., and Polaschek, D. L. L. (2005). Do child molesters deliberately fake good on cognitive distortion questionnaires? An information processing based investigation. Sexual Abuse: *A Journal of Research and Treatment*, 183-200.

Gannon, T. A., Polaschek, D. L. L., and Ward T. (2005). Social cognition and sexual offenders. In M. McMurran and J. McGuire (Eds.), *Social problem solving and offenders.* (pp. 223-247). Chichester, UK: Wiley.

Gannon, T. A., Ward, T., and Collie, R. (2006). Cognitive Distortions in Child Molesters: Theoretical and Research Developments over the Past Two Decades. *Manuscript submitted for publication.*

Gannon, T. A., Wright, D. B., Beech, A. R. and Williams, S. A. (2006). Do child molesters have cognitive distortions? What does their memory recall tell us? *Journal of Sexual Aggression*, 12, 5-18.

Garner D. M., and Bemis K. M. (1982). A cognitive-behavioral approach to anorexia nervosa. *Cognitive Therapy and Research*. 6, 123-50.

Gray, N. S., Brown, A. S., MacCulloch, M. J., Smith, J., and Snowden, R. J. (2005). An implicit test of the association between children and sex in pedophiles. *Journal of Abnormal Psychology*, 114, 304-308.

Greenwald, A. G., McGhee, J. L., and Schwartz, J. L. (1998). Measuring individual difference in implicit cognition: The Implicit Association Test. *Journal of Personality and Social Psychology*, 74, 1464-1480.

Hall, G. C. N., and Hirschman, R. (1992). Sexual aggression against children: A conceptual perspective of etiology. *Criminal Justice and Behaviour*, 19, 8-23.

Hayashino, D. S., Wurtele, S. K., and Klebe, K. J. (1995). Child molesters: An examination of cognitive factors. *Journal of Interpersonal Violence*, 10, 106-116.

Hollon, S. D., and Kriss, M. R. (1984). Cognitive factors in clinical research and practice. *Clinical Psychology Review*, 4, 35-76.

Hsu, L. M., Santelli, J., and Hsu, J. R. (1989). Faking detection validity and increment validity of response latencies to MMPI subtle and obvious items. *Journal of Personality Assessment*, 53, 278-295.

Langevin, R. (1991). A note on the problem of response set in measuring cognitive distortions. *Annals of Sex Research*, 4, 287-292.

Mann, R. E., and Beech, A. R. (2003). Cognitive distortions, schemas, and implicit theories. In T. Ward, D. R. Laws, and S. M. Hudson (Eds.), *Sexual deviance: Issues and controversies* (pp. 135-153). Thousand Oaks, CA: Sage.

Mann, R. E., and Shingler, J. (2006). Schema-driven cognition in sexual offenders: theory, assessment and treatment. In W. L. Marshall, Y. M. Fernandez, L. E. Marshall, and G. A. Serran (Eds.), *Sexual offender treatment: Controversial issues* (pp. 173-185). Chichester, UK: Wiley.

Marshall, W. L., Marshall, L. E., Sachdav, S., and Kruger, R. (2003). Distorted attitudes and perceptions, and their relationship with self esteem and coping in child molesters. *Sexual Abuse: A Journal of Research and Treatment*, 15, 171-181.

Maruna, S., and Mann, R. (in press). A fundamental attribution error? Rethinking cognitive distortions. *Legal and Criminological Psychology.*

Marziano, V., Ward., T., Beech, A. R., and Pattison, R. (2005). Identification of five fundamental implicit theories underlying cognitive distortions in child abusers: A preliminary study. *Psychology, Crime and Law*, 12, 97-105.

McGrath, M. L., Cann, S., and Konopasky, R. J. (1998). New measures of defensiveness, empathy, and cognitive distortions for sexual offenders against children. *Sexual Abuse: A Journal of Research and Treatment, 10,* 25-36.

McGuire, J. (2001). What works in correctional intervention? Evidence and practical implications. In G. Bernfeld, A. W. Leschied, and D. P. Farrington, (Eds.), *Offender rehabilitation in action: Implementing and evaluating effective programs* (pp. 25-43). London: Wiley.

Mihailides, S., Devilly, G. J., and Ward, T. (2004). Implicit cognitive distortions and sexual offending. *Sexual Abuse: A Journal of Research and Treatment, 16*, 333-350.

Murphy, W. D. (1990). Assessment and modification of cognitive distortions in sex offenders. In W. L. Marshall, D. R. Laws, and Barbaree (Eds.), *Handbook of sexual assault:Issues, theories, and treatment of the offender* (pp. 331-342). NY: Plenum.

Neidigh, L., and Krop, H. (1992). Cognitive distortions among child sexual offenders. *Journal of Sex Education and Therapy, 18,* 208-215.

Pollock, N. L., and Hashmall, J. M. (1991).The excuses of child molesters. *Behavioral Sciences and the Law, 9,* 53-59.

Rachman, S., and Shafran, R. (1999). Cognitive distortions: Thought-action fusion. *Clinical Psychology and Psychotherapy, 6*, 80-85.

Salkovskis, P. M. (1985). Obsessional-compulsive problems: A cognitive behavioural analysis. *Behaviour Research and Therapy, 23,* 571 - 583

Saradjian, A., and Nobus, D. (2003). Cognitive distortions of religious professionals who sexually abuse children. *Journal of Interpersonal Violence, 18,* 905-923.

Sherman, S. J., Judd, C. M., and Park, B. (1989). Social cognition. *Annual Review of Psychology, 40,* 281-326.

Stermac, L., and Segal, Z. (1989). Adult sexual contact with children: An examination of cognitive factors. *Behavior Therapy, 20,* 573-584.

Thompson D. A., Berg K. M., and Shatford L. A. (1987) The heterogeneity of bulimic symptomatology: cognitive and behavioral dimensions. *International Journal of Eating Disorders, 6,* 215 - 234.

Thornton, D., and Shingler, J. (2001). *Impact of schema level work on sexual offenders' cognitive distortions.* Paper presented at the 20th Annual Research and Treatment Conference for the Treatment of Sexual Abusers, San Antonio, USA.

Tierney, D. W., and McCabe, M. P. (2001). An evaluation of self-report measures of cognitive distortions and empathy among Australian sex offenders. *Archives of Sexual Behavior, 30*, 495-519.

Vanhouche, W., and Vertommen, H., (1999). Assessing cognitive distortions in sex offenders: A review of commonly used versus recently developed instruments. *Psychologica Belgica, 39*, 163-187.

Ward, T. (2000). Sexual offenders' cognitive distortions as implicit theories. *Aggression and Violent Behavior, 5*, 491-507.

Ward, T., Gannon, T. A., and Keown, K. (2006). Beliefs, values, and action: The judgment model of cognitive distortions. *Aggression and Violent Behavior: A Review Journal, 11,* 323-340.

Ward, T., Hudson, S. M, Johnston, L., and Marshall, W. L. (1997). Cognitive distortions in sex offenders: An integrative review. *Clinical Psychology Review, 17*, 479-507.

Ward, T., and Keenan, T. (1999). Child molesters' implicit theories. *Journal of Interpersonal Violence, 14,* 821-838.

Ward, T., and Siegert, R. (2002). Toward a comprehensive theory of child sexual abuse: A Theory knitting perspective. *Psychology, Crime, and Law, 8*, 319-351.

INDEX

B

C

D

F

G

H

I

N

O

P

Q

R

S

T

U

V

W

Y